HABIT THAT!

HABIT THAT!

HOW YOU CAN HEALTH UP IN JUST 5 MINUTES A DAY

JAIME HOPE, MD

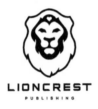

LIONCREST
PUBLISHING

HABIT THAT!

How You Can Health Up in Just 5 Minutes a Day

ISBN 978-1-5445-1262-4 *Hardcover*

978-1-5445-1261-7 *Paperback*

978-1-5445-1260-0 *Ebook*

978-1-5445-1303-4 *Audiobook*

For Bobbie

CONTENTS

INTRODUCTION 9

PART I: FROM MOTIVATION TO MOMENTUM

1. WHY YOUR *REAL WHY* MATTERS MOST.......................37

2. OBSTACLES AND MOTIVATION..................................65

3. WORK SMARTER, NOT HARDER...............................97

PART II: THE FOUR PILLARS OF HEALTH

4. EAT.. 129

5. SLEEP... 181

6. BURN...227

7. RELEASE... 269

CONCLUSION 315

APPENDIX A: FIVE-MINUTE HEALTH-UPS 329

APPENDIX B: THE 12 REASONS EXERCISE..................347

APPENDIX C: THE SMARTER GOALS WORKSHEET.... 351

APPENDIX D: TRACKING YOUR FITNESS GOALS.......355

APPENDIX E: IDENTIFYING YOUR WEAKEST LEG 357

ACKNOWLEDGMENTS....................................... 369

ABOUT THE AUTHOR... 381

INTRODUCTION

TAKE ONE STEP

If you read all of the popular books and take the advice of all of the gurus of the minute, it's easier than ever to live healthy nowadays! You simply have to check off the following boxes every single day:

☐ Spend an hour practicing yoga.

☐ Spend an hour exercising.

☐ Spend an hour meditating.

☐ Buy all organic foods and spend a couple hours crafting those overpriced ingredients into a perfectly balanced meal. Aaannnddd...don't forget the thirty minutes it takes to make those green smoothies every day.

- ☐ Make sure you have some downtime for staring out the window with a cup of tea.
- ☐ Get eight to ten hours of sleep every night.

Oh, by the way, I almost forgot. You also need to:

- ☐ Work hard at your job to get ahead.
- ☐ Spend hours of quality time building meaningful and connected relationships with friends and family.
- ☐ Take care of all those daily chores around the house. (That laundry isn't going to fold itself, you know.)

Exhausted yet? Discouraged? Bewildered? Kind of sore from pulling a hamstring trying to do the "bird of paradise" yoga pose whilst chopping your organic kale?

You don't have to be a math whiz to realize all the time it takes to practice all the magical healthy life hacks, which add up to more than twenty-four hours of "healthy living" each day. We all want to do the right thing, but the right thing often feels impossible, doesn't it?

WHO HAS THE TIME?

Wouldn't it be great if life came with a great big pause button, like a Zack Morris time-out on *Saved by the Bell*?[1]

---

1   Don't tell Mr. Belding I'm making *Saved by the Bell* references. I don't want to end up in the principal's office—again!

You could put your work and personal life on hold, decide what healthy choices you wanted to make, put them into action, and then carry on with your new healthy life! As great as that would be, so far I've found that life doesn't work that way.

Healthy choices have to be made within the realistic context of our busy lives. The tricky part is that circumstances are always changing. Living healthy may be easy at certain points in your life, but at other points, it's a chattering monkey mocking you from the sidelines. My friend—let's call her Lucy—has experienced plenty of ups and downs on the road to healthy living, as these three snapshots taken along her health journey demonstrate.

SNAPSHOT #1

Lucy is the outdoorsy type. She's always loved being active, but lately other aspects of her life are taking up increasingly more time. Her career is taking off, which is great, but success has a way of bringing added pressure. On top of that, she and her husband recently began divorce proceedings. Now, even when she has time to get outside for a day hike, she usually isn't in the mood. Perhaps it's best to just put her active life on hold until everything else blows over.

SNAPSHOT #2

Lucy has spent the past few years building a family with her new spouse. It's been a great few years, but if Lucy is being honest, she has yet to resume that active life she put on hold so long ago. She has gained more weight than she'd care to admit, and the lack of proper diet and activity has started to take a mental toll. Enough is enough, she decides. It's time to change. The next week, Lucy goes all in. With the support of her spouse, she commits to a new gym and personal trainer, makes daycare arrangements for her kids, and starts counting calories to speed up her weight loss. In six months, she's at her target weight and feeling great.

SNAPSHOT #3

Lucy isn't the four-days-a-week gym warrior she used to be. She values that six-month span where she went all out for her goals, but as a working mother, she knew it wasn't sustainable over the long term—and she's okay with that. These days, she's health-conscious but practical. She goes to the gym twice a week and makes sure to eat plenty of fruits and veggies, but she also doesn't feel any guilt for taking time off from exercise now and then and allowing herself the occasional Pepsi. She knows she could do more, but these are the habits that fit with her life right now, and she feels like she's found a good balance.

LIVE FOR TODAY (AND FOR TOMORROW)

Sometimes Lucy couldn't find five minutes a day for healthy habits. Other times, Lucy wanted to reach a goal so badly that she went all in to make it possible. Now, she's somewhere in-between, active but not overzealous, food-conscious but not diet-crazy. It took a while to get there, but these days Lucy feels balanced.

That's how I want you to feel, too.

Wherever you are on your own health journey, whether you are a beginner or begin-againer, that's a great starting point. Be happy with who you are and where you are right now. Whoever you are and wherever you're starting from, I'm here to meet you there and help you get a little better each day.

HEALTHY LIVING SHOULDN'T BE INTIMIDATING

This isn't a book about fad diets, quick fixes, or crazy weight loss schemes. Actually, it's not specifically about weight loss at all, though that is often a wonderful by-product of healthy living.

Instead, it's about creating long-term well-being through small, sustained daily efforts. If you have five minutes a day, you have time to create a healthy habit.

IT'S ALL ABOUT THE QUICK WINS

Everybody wants to follow the miracle all-bacon diet that will somehow make them a happy, well-rested, stress-free triathlete in a month's time. I'd love to tell you that's a viable, scientifically backed option. It would have saved me a lot of time writing this book!

But seriously, if you're looking for the quick fix, then I recommend signing up for the Bullshit of the Month Club. Here's how you join: go to a bookstore, close your eyes, and throw a dart in the fad diet book section. Whatever that dart hits, pick up that gem of a book, and then follow it. Mostly likely, you *will* lose weight...temporarily. Then, you will gain it all back again when you get off the diet and return to real life (sound familiar?).

However, if you are sick of the yo-yo world of fancy-named-but-ill-conceived fake diet plans, then I've got a new club for you: the Habit That Club! Here in the Habit That Club, it's all about creating good habits and playing the long game. Yes, it's true that the long game can be intimidating, especially if you feel like you need to change everything about your lifestyle all at once. Don't worry; I get it. The long game scares away a lot of people.

Not you, though. No way. You picked up this book because you're ready for something different. You're here right now because you came here for *real* answers and *real* results, not some false, fleeting overnight success story. The good news, though, is you don't have to choose between quick wins and long-term success. You can have both!

I'm a big fan of quick wins. We all are. That's just how our minds work. There's nothing better than checking off a box on our to-do lists and feeling like we accomplished something, no matter how fleeting it might have been. So, I'm thinking that rather than let our desire for quick wins derail us, why don't we use this impulse to our advantage in service of our long-term goals?

For years now, I've used quick wins to anchor my healthy living journey. It all began with a simple daily task: drink more water. The goal was simple, but it also felt real and attainable. Every day I met my water quota felt like a victory, like I controlled my own destiny. (Cue the superhero background music.)

Soon I wanted to do more. One day I added flossing to my routine. Then I focused on eating better by replacing my usual grazing food—Cheetos and M&M's—with fruits and veggies. With each new habit, I gave my brain the quick wins and sense of accomplishment it wanted, all while setting my body up for long-term success. And if a picky-eater-junk-food-junkie like me can do it, then you can, too.

Imagine you and your friend decided to do 1,825 sit-ups last year. But while you focused on doing five sit-ups every day, your friend tried to take care of all 1,825 on New Year's Eve. Who do you think actually reached that sit-up goal, you or your friend? All other things being equal, whose body do you think is going to look better?

Mostly likely, your friend didn't reach her goal. Even if she did, putting everything off to the last minute probably didn't make much of a difference for her body—other than leaving her super sore and exhausted for a couple days. That's not how our bodies find balance.

Since you focused on five sit-ups every day, on the other hand, you're feeling a world of difference. Why? Because your junior high math teacher was right all those years ago when you were learning about compounding interest—small, sustained efforts *do* add up over time. Just like a penny invested each day in a compounding savings account builds up to huge financial returns over your lifetime, a quick win invested in your health savings account each day is going to add up to a lifetime of good health— and the more tiny deposits you make over time, the more interest you accrue!

A LITTLE ABOUT ME

If you picked up this book, it means you're interested in a healthier lifestyle. I think I can help, too—and I'm excited to guide you through the Habit That process! But first, let me tell you who I am and why I wrote this book.

Medicine has been a part of my life for more than a dozen years. For much of that time, I've worked as an ER doctor outside of Detroit, Michigan, in one of the busiest emergency departments in the country. I've seen things most people can't even imagine. Many of the people who come in for help are having the worst day of their life. No one wants to be there, and some of them don't make it out. The sad truth is, with healthier habits, many of them wouldn't *need* to be there in the first place.

I wrote this book to help people like you stay happy, healthy, and out of the ER. I'm going to show you a lot of ways to do this, but that doesn't mean you have to try every single one. Living healthy doesn't have to be so complicated. If you have five minutes to build a healthy habit, then you have time to make a positive impact on your life. Five minutes are better than no minutes!

I want your health span to be as long as your life-span. I love my job, but if I can help the world get so healthy that I end up out of work, that would be the most amazing day of my life.

WHY DID I BECOME A DOCTOR?

From the time I was a little kid, I always thought it would be so cool to be a doctor. My pediatrician used to do goofy things, like taking my long hair and putting it on his bald head, just to make us kids laugh. I toyed around with other possible future occupations as I grew up—teacher, astronaut, journalist, marine biologist, Fly Girl on *In Living Color*—but the idea of being a doctor always stuck with me. I realized I wanted to be a doctor when I was around ten years old and my BFF fell off the trampoline and fracture-dislocated her elbow. I remember looking at her arm, bent in a way it wasn't supposed to bend, thinking I might be able to fix it. I certainly wanted to try! Wisely, she wouldn't let me.

Years later, I was a first-generation college student. The road to doctorhood wasn't always easy, but the more I learned about medicine, the more I loved it—*all* of it. In fact, it took me forever to settle on a specialty because everything seemed so interesting.

When I rotated into the emergency department, suddenly everything clicked. There, I performed all kinds of procedures on all kinds of people with all kinds of maladies. I took care of infants, children, adults, and elderly patients alike, and I loved it.

Being an ER doctor is the coolest, most amazing privilege.

I get to help people through incredibly trying moments. In the process, I learn some remarkable details about their lives, their fears, their hopes, and their dreams.

Does being a doctor have some drawbacks? You bet. The emergency department is open 24/7/365, so I sometimes work weekends, nights, and holidays. The ER, as you can imagine, isn't the most relaxing place. On top of that, people always worry about the way they eat in front of me—especially after I became an out-and-proud health nut. I've had coworkers literally hide their lunch from me in the break room.

Trust me, I'm not here to judge. I don't care what you had for lunch today (though I *do* hope you enjoyed it). I'm just here to offer some advice on how to build a few practical, real-world habits—and then stick to them.

My #1 Goal: Extending Your Health Span

If there's one thing I've learned through my interactions in the ER, as an assistant professor, or as a professional speaker, it's that many of us are putting off healthy living for later.

It's almost like we're all waiting for this magical Utopian moment where we have tons of free time, tons of money, and tons of motivation to take care of our health. I hate to be the bearer of bad news, but that magical moment is never going to come. In fact, if you wait for it too long, your health span may be over before your life-span.

I understand you're legitimately busy in your life. I also understand that you *do* want to live healthier, but too often you find yourself stuck looking for a path forward. My number one goal is to extend your health span by helping you find that path forward.

Getting and staying on that path begins with a little shift in mindset. When it comes to healthy living, most of us focus on where we want to be in magical Utopia, not where we are *right now*. I say take the opposite approach. Look at where you are today, decide where you want to be at the end of the month, and come up with a few practical quick wins to get you there. You may never find Utopia (I still haven't), but you will find a happier, healthier life along the way.

NERD ALERTS

If you couldn't tell by now, I'm a little goofy and a lot passionate.

Science fascinates me. I'm required to keep learning for my job, but even in my free time, I'm constantly reading up on subjects like metabolic physiology, the endocrine system, human behavior change, personal development, and even business development.

Yes indeed, I'm a huge nerd, and I couldn't be happier about it.

The bottom line, though, is it doesn't matter how much I know if you can't relate. I wrote this book to help *you*, and that means I'll be putting aside the nerd speak—mostly. Sometimes I can't help but throw down and geek out on some science.

Throughout this book, you're going to see plenty of "nerd alerts" where I do exactly that. It's okay to skip them if you choose, but anytime you want to unleash your own inner nerd, I'm happy to oblige.

FOUR PATIENTS, FOUR JOURNEYS

To help guide you through this book, I've created four patients whose journeys we will follow in each chapter. Though fictional, these four avatars are conglomerates of the real people I've encountered in my job. After all, I haven't met just a few people worried about finding the time for healthy habits. I've met thousands.

Each of these patients is struggling to make healthier choices within the context of their daily life. Each is struggling with one or more of the four pillars of health (more on those in just a moment). Each is struggling with finding the kind of balance it took my friend Lucy years to find.

As we move through their journeys, keep in mind that, just like us, none of them is going to find Utopia. None of them is going to dramatically change how they live and become a healthy-living spokesperson. Instead, these patients are going to model small, practical, and real-world adjustments to their daily lives, demonstrating the compounding effect of committing to one healthy habit at a time.

You're going to learn all about our new friends in the following chapters. For now, here's a little background to help you understand who they are and where they came from.

Sarah the "Sandwich Generation" Mother

At thirty-two, Sarah has her hands full taking care of her three rambunctious (but amazing) children, ages two, four, and seven. She used to get some help from her parents, but as they've aged, they've become more dependent on their daughter than she has on them, making Sarah a full-fledged member of the "Sandwich Generation." With a full-time job to boot, Sarah often feels overwhelmed by all her responsibilities, looking after everyone's health but her own, especially when it comes to her eating habits.

Bill the Burned-Out Entrepreneur

This forty-five-year-old entrepreneur worked his whole life to get where he is today, and he's damn proud of the business he's built from the ground up. Unfortunately, decades of burning the candles at both ends have left Bill not feeling like himself. Putting the world on his shoulders every day has left him stressed and exhausted, but he isn't sure what he can do to change.

Mary the Empty Nester

At fifty-six, Mary just watched her youngest move off to college, and for the first time in decades, she has no one to worry about but herself. Now that her kids are spreading their wings and forging lives of their own, Mary has been given an opportunity to rediscover herself. She's not in the best shape, but she's not in the worst, either. She wants to make her remaining thirty or forty years count, perhaps even run a charity 5K race, but even when she exercises, she has no energy, and she can't figure out why.

George the Retiree with a Bum Knee

Now retired and living on a fixed income, this sixty-eight-year-old plumber has had a good and fulfilling life so far. George has always found great pleasure in his work, which has allowed him to keep both his body and his mind occupied. Despite this, years of unhealthy eating habits are catching up to him, and a recent knee surgery made him realize he's no spring chicken anymore. His doctor told him that if he doesn't start taking a little weight off, his other knee—and possibly his hips—will need surgery next. George knows it's time to turn off the TV, get out of his recliner, and start moving around, but what can a guy with a bum knee do?

SUDDENLY...A MUFFIN

I love memes. I use them in my talks all the time, and I'll be quoting some of my favorites throughout this book. One of my favorites is a picture of a giant muffin crushing a car. Beneath the photo, the caption reads,

"Suddenly...a muffin."

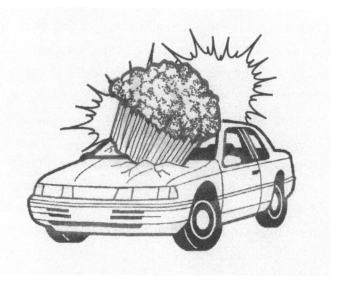

We all experience muffin moments in our lives, those times where disaster seems to just drop out of the sky and change everything.

I've certainly had plenty of my own. A couple years ago, I had settled into a great, healthy routine with my kids, when suddenly...a muffin—my mother-in-law was diagnosed with pancreatic cancer. This shocking news and the full-time healthcare support my mother-in-law needed altered my routines in a big way. It was an honor to be her care-giver, however, and I soon learned to create a new normal during the two blessed years we had while she gracefully progressed through this final, trying stage of her life.

When I sat down to write this book, suddenly...another muffin—some nagging abdominal pain that led to a surprise emergency appendectomy! Forget that perfectly planned publishing schedule and everything else I had going on. My body had other plans, and, although we doctors don't always make the greatest patients, I was forced to shut my ambitious agenda down for a little bit.

Chances are, you've experienced your share of muffin moments, too. And chances are, more muffin moments are waiting in your future—just as they're waiting for Sarah, Bill, Mary, and George in the chapters ahead.

Muffins happen. That's how real life works. Whether it's a medical emergency or a move to a new town, a big routine-changing event is going to happen.

When that event comes, I want you to be ready for it. By building a life focused on good habits and quick wins, you *will be*.

THE TWO PARTS OF THIS BOOK

If there's one idea you take away from this book, it's that if you only have five minutes to spare every day, you have enough time to practice healthy habits.

This leads to a couple questions. First, how do you set actionable goals and create sustainable habits? Second, if you do only have five minutes a day for healthy habits, what should you focus on? Well, as luck would have it, I've divided the book into two parts specifically to help you master these two elements of healthy living.

PART I: FROM MOTIVATION TO MOMENTUM

We usually think of habits in negative terms, such as biting your nails or smoking. However, the truth is that you can form *good* habits, too.

The road to a healthy lifestyle *begins* with proper motivation, but motivation alone won't sustain you forever. Motivation takes both emotional and cognitive effort, and you don't want to be in a position where the fickle tides of motivation are the only resource you have. The trick is to stay motivated long enough for that effort to become a habit, which is an automatic behavior that's much easier to sustain. When that happens, the rest is easy.

That's what Part I of this book is all about: turning motivation into healthy habits. Chapters 1 through 3 will introduce three essential tools:

1. Finding your *real why*
2. Identifying and navigating obstacles to starting and sustaining your healthy habits
3. Turning your *real why* into everyday habits by setting SMARTER Goals

These practices form the foundation on which the four pillars of health, Part II of the book, will stand. After all, it's one thing to want to eat, sleep, burn, and release better, but without the tools laid out in Part I, you might not know where to start.

PART II: THE FOUR PILLARS OF HEALTH

Imagine everything in your life that's important to you—your family, your friends, your relationships, your career, your goals, your habits, and your dreams—all piled up on a table.

Holding up this table are the four legs of your life-sustaining practices: diet, rest, exercise, and stress management.

The strength of each leg depends on how well you manage them. If you ignore one leg, your table might be a little wobbly, but it's still doing its job.

However, if you start ignoring a second leg—or a third (or a fourth!)—your table is in trouble. You simply won't be able to hold up all those wonderful aspects of your life anymore.

Part II of this book is all about strengthening your table so nothing slips off. Each chapter will focus on a different leg: eat (proper diet), sleep (good rest), burn (exercise), and release (stress). By building the strongest table you can, you'll learn to not merely survive, but *thrive*.

Some pillars are going to resonate with you more than others. However, as you read through them, it's important you keep two things in mind:

1. You need all four pillars to be a healthy person.
2. The pillar you need to work on the most might not be what you think. For instance, you can't lose weight if you're full of anxiety (seriously, your body won't let you). If you focus on one pillar at the expense of another, you probably won't see the progress you were hoping for.

Once you've read through each chapter, you'll get a quiz to help you identify your weakest leg. Then, using the goal-setting strategies of Part I, you can start building the healthy habits necessary for a strong, sturdy table.

FIVE-MINUTE HEALTH-UPS

One of my primary motivators in writing this is to help people understand that living healthy can be as simple as pre-chopping vegetables on a Sunday evening, taking a brief walk around the block, or taking five minutes to relax and clear your mind in the middle of a busy day. As you'll hear me say time and again in this book, if you only have five minutes, you have time to health up, to take one step forward with your mind and body, and boost your baseline. Five minutes is better than no minutes.

To show you how easy those five-minute health-up opportunities can be, I've included tons of useful examples in Appendix A, as well as in the context of our four patients at the end of each chapter in Part II. Some of these are practices I've incorporated into my own life, and others are suggestions I've received from friends, family, and patients. While these examples are far from the final word on the subject, they should give you a better idea of how you can grab hold of those many small opportunities in your day and use that time to create a healthier, happier you!

To get a sense of what works for you as you learn ways to create and strengthen your healthy pathways, I encourage you to try them all out. Whatever helps you the most, keep doing—and if you'd like, you can even spend more than five minutes on them! For bonus points, try creating your own five-minute (or any amount of time!) activities and share them with other people on a journey similar to yours on our Habit That Tribe Facebook page.

THERE'S A DIFFERENCE BETWEEN "SURVIVAL" AND "OPTIMAL"

In case you didn't know already, your body is amazing. It's exquisitely designed to survive nearly anything—from famine to running from a bear, and everything in-between. You can survive on booze and doughnuts for quite a while. You can survive for a long time if you're sleep-deprived and stressed out. You can even survive for a while if all you do is sit around watching reruns of *Matlock*, like our friend George does.

Just know this: there is a big difference between "survival" and "optimal."

People often equate healthy living with diet first, and exercise second. Those help, but not if you sacrifice sleep and mental health in the process. Fad diets and exercise gadgets promote quick fixes. It's easy to see their appeal, but they rarely translate into long-term health gains. When we follow these fads, we may think we're doing ourselves a favor, but we're still only surviving.

This book isn't about survival living. It's about *optimal* living. It's about finding a healthy set point so you feel good, so you feel stable, so you feel *balanced*.

The medical term for this is *homeostasis*, and it's different for everybody. Some people are going to be naturally thin, even if they aren't eating healthy, while others are going to carry a little bit of fat even if they're making healthy choices. We'll be talking about weight loss in this book, but only in the service of healthy living.

That's where the long-term lifestyle comes in. As a very wise person once said, "A person who is healthy has a thousand wishes. A person who is unhealthy has only one."[2] What's the one wish? To be healthy.

Survival is not enough. One wish is not enough. I want you to have as many wishes as you please throughout the rest of your happy, healthy life.

DO I WANT TO HABIT THAT?

We are creatures of habit. It's human nature, and there's no sense fighting it. Sometimes, those habits are beneficial, like how you always make sure to brush your teeth twice a day. Other times, they're not doing you much good, like when you catch yourself mindlessly snacking on M&M's immediately after lunch.

---

2   Which wise person said that? According to Google, this saying either came from author A. G. Riddle or an old Indian proverb. It could be either, or it could be neither. This is why I always tell patients not to take web-based symptom checkers too seriously. No matter what Dr. Google says, whatever's bothering you is probably not cancer, and you're probably not dying. That said, it's always better to err on the side of caution and see a doctor whenever you're concerned about your health or well-being. And take everything you read on the internet with a grain of salt.

Here's the cool part: our habits don't control us. *We control our habits.* We get to pick which behaviors we want to emphasize and which ones we want to let go. That's what the Habit That lifestyle is all about: embracing the idea that our human tendency toward habit-making can be used for *good*—and taking an active role in the habits we create. Rather than teaching you to resist your natural impulses toward quick wins and easy habits, I'm going to teach you how to use them to your advantage by creating daily behaviors you can be proud of.

As we get ready to push forward into Part I, I want you to take a look at all your daily routines—good, bad, and anything in-between. Maybe you like to walk a quick lap around the block after lunch, or maybe you always graze on beef jerky around two o'clock.

With each routine you identify, ask yourself one question: "Do I want to habit that?"

If you do want to habit that behavior, then by all means keep at it. However, if you don't want to habit that, then read on!

PART I

—

FROM MOTIVATION TO MOMENTUM

CHAPTER 1

WHY YOUR *REAL* *WHY* MATTERS MOST

New Year's Day is the most magical day of the year. On this day, we're the best versions of ourselves, living our best lives. "This is going to be my year!" we declare, but by December 31, we're left looking back at the year that just passed, scratching our heads, and wondering what happened to all those ambitious New Year's plans.

"Maybe I overshot a little," we say, "but this next year really *is* going to be my year!" Then we sit down, cross out the previous year's resolutions, and proceed to write out an almost identical set of new goals.[3] If we're using

---

3   Fun footnote: The top ten most common resolutions are: exercise more, lose weight, get organized, learn something new/take a class, spend less money, quit smoking, spend more time with loved ones, eat healthier, travel more, and read more. There is some variation depending on which survey and which year it is, but these are the perennial favorites.

the same piece of paper each year, it might end up looking something like this:

NEW YEAR'S RESOLUTIONS FOR ~~2016~~ ~~2017~~ ~~2018~~ 2019

1. Lose ~~more~~ weight (again)
2. Get fit (next year)
3. ~~Give up alcohol and cigarettes.~~ Drink less.
4. ~~Stand up to boss.~~ Find job.
5. ~~Be nicer~~ Try to be nicer to my ~~wife~~ ex-wife.
6. Sort out junk in ~~shed~~ life.

What's going on here? What is this cruel trick of human nature? Why, oh why, do so many of us fail to live up to our goals each year?

"I can't believe it's been a year since I didn't become a better person!"

Well, the simple answer is that we're not really setting goals. Instead, we're making wishes. I *wish* I could be nicer to my spouse. I *wish* I could drink less. I *wish* I could spend less money.

It doesn't matter how motivated you feel on New Year's Day. If all you've got is a vague goal-wish without a concrete plan for action, you're going to find it pretty hard to follow through over the course of the year.

LET'S TALK MOTIVATION

Author Zig Ziglar has a great way of looking at the motivation conundrum. "Motivation isn't permanent," he says, "but neither is bathing." This puts motivation in a much more real-world context. It's not a matter of having the willpower to get up and make a healthy choice once. It's a matter of creating and committing to habits that you can repeat *every day*. You can't bathe once on New Year's Day and expect to be clean for the whole year! To that end, here are a few things to keep in mind.

THERE'S NO MAGIC MOMENT

"Tomorrow (noun): A mystical land where 99 percent of all human productivity, motivation, and achievement is stored."

Wouldn't it be great if it only took one magical day—perhaps New Year's Day, perhaps tomorrow, perhaps next Monday—to get healthy? All you'd have to do is make a wish, and then suddenly, you would look and feel better than a million bucks.

At the risk of sounding like the obvious police, that's not going to happen. A one-time declaration does not make a healthy person. If you're part of the New Year's resolution crowd, you probably realize this by about January fifth, and then you spend the rest of the year beating yourself up for your failure to live up to your goal. I don't know about you, but that sounds like a lousy mood to be in for the majority of the year.

MOTIVATION IS TEMPORARY, HABITS ARE PERMANENT

"Motivation get you going. Habit keeps you there."

—ZIG ZIGLAR

Real motivation isn't about finding that magic, life-changing moment. In fact, the whole idea of motivation isn't that sustainable. If you're like me, some days you feel like you can take on the world, while other days are a struggle not to put your pants on inside-out.

So here's the question: on those other days when you're not feeling super motivated, how can you be expected to make healthy choices?

Well, what do you do when you don't feel like brushing your teeth? I bet you brush them anyway—and even if you don't that day, I bet you brush them extra the next day.

Have you ever stopped to think about why that is, why

you keep brushing your teeth almost every day, no matter what mood you're in?

The answer is that you formed a habit, and once you did, you didn't have to think about brushing your teeth anymore. Repeat any activity long enough, and it will become a habit. When it does, it's a big weight off your cognitive load. In other words, if you don't have to think about your habit, if it becomes automatic, then you're free to think about other things—like building off your success and forming another good habit!

DON'T WAIT FOR MOTIVATION

All this is to say that if you're waiting to feel motivated before acting on your health goals, then you're doing it backward. I know it sounds counterintuitive, but bear with me on this.

Have you ever had one of those days where you knew you needed to go to the gym, had zero motivation to do so, but ended up going anyway? How did you feel afterward? Pretty good, right?

Healthy living isn't about motivation. It's about committing. If you spend all your time waiting until you *feel* like eating more servings of fruits and vegetables, you might never make them a part of your daily habits.

Do the actions, do the habit, and the good feelings will follow. With each little win, it gets easier to keep your promise the next time. Eventually the habit takes hold, and you'll be mad about the days you *can't* perform the healthy habit—be it eating your veggies, going to the gym, getting enough sleep, or taking a mindfulness break. It would be like somebody stealing all the toothbrushes from your house.

Here's another way to look at the Habit That lifestyle: imagine you're sledding down a snow-covered hill. The more you perform the action, the more you start to carve deeper paths into the snow on the hill. The first few runs, you coast directionless down the side of the mountain, but eventually, you start carving out a set path in the snow, freeing you to think less about controlling your trajectory and more about how much fun you're having. Each time you repeat a healthy habit, you strengthen and deepen that pathway. That's how you Habit That!

Years ago, my dad carved his own Habit That tracks by committing to going to the gym three times a week, without fail. When his gym changed owners and he didn't care for the new environment, he didn't give up the habit. He simply found a new gym where he could continue his habit. Similarly, I read about an author who carved his Habit That tracks by designating different coffee shops and work environments for different days of the week, each associated with a unique productive activity.

FINDING YOUR *REAL WHY*

Have you ever thought about why you brush your teeth? Is it because they feel gross if you don't? Is it because you're afraid of tooth decay? Is it because you like having a nice set of pearly whites when you smile?

Whatever the reason, that's your *real why* for brushing your teeth. It's what keeps you going even on those nights when you're feeling so drained or lazy that you want to skip brushing entirely and head straight to bed.

For every good habit you want to build, you need to find your *real why*. The *real why* itself can be just about anything. Maybe you want your butt to look good in your favorite pair of jeans. Maybe you want to walk around the block without feeling winded, or maybe you want enough energy to keep up with your kids every day. Whatever the case, your *real why* reminds you of the big picture and propels you forward when motivation fails.

ABSTRACT *WHYS* HELP NO ONE

I'm certainly not the first person to talk about finding your *why*. Most of my patients are already familiar with the idea when I bring it up. If I ask them why they want to quit smoking, they might reply that they don't want to get black lung or cancer.

The fear of black lung or lung cancer may be sufficient motivation for some people—particularly if someone in their lives was diagnosed with it—but often, when I hear a smoker say this, I wonder if they're just telling me what I want to hear as a doctor. *Every* smoker is aware of these risks. The warning is right there on every pack of cigarettes. If the warning on the pack alone deterred people, then nobody would smoke.

Finding your *real why* for healthy living is no different. An abstract awareness of lung cancer may contribute to a desire to quit, but usually there's a deeper reason that's much more personal, that you might even be embarrassed to share with others. Similarly, saying "I want to get healthy" or "I want to get thinner" is a great start, and probably true, but it likely won't resonate enough with you to build new, sustainable habits when the Netflix and snack binges beckon. It's too abstract, too detached from your everyday experiences to resonate with you. And if it doesn't resonate with you, then you won't do it.

GET SPECIFIC

I often joke that being a doctor—especially an ER doctor— is a lot like speed dating. You come into my ER, and in three minutes, I'm going to have you naked and telling me personal details about your life.

My patients must trust me as quickly as possible. If I make them feel uncomfortable or embarrassed, they might leave out vital information, which in turn could lead to a misdiagnosis or a missed problem altogether.

Because I focus on creating a comfortable environment, my patients share some pretty personal information. Often, some element of this information, whether it's their hopes, their fears, or their insecurities, becomes the kernel of their *real why*—their true motivation for making a change and choosing a healthier lifestyle.

For instance, one of my patients realized he had to lose weight while he was on a flight to a business conference. He literally couldn't fit comfortably into his seat and had to ask the flight attendant for a seat belt extender. He *hated* that feeling. He told me he had never been more embarrassed than at that moment. Keeping that experience from happening again became his *real why*.

Your *real why* should be just as specific and just as personal. It may even be just as uncomfortable. If you get nervous and sweaty thinking about it, if you feel embarrassed sharing it with others, odds are you've found a *why* that's real and authentic.

I'm all for setting ambitious goals. If you want to be a marathon runner, then I want you to work toward that goal. In fact, I'm going to spend all of Chapter 3 talking about how to set SMARTER Goals to ensure your success.

That said, having your eyes on the finish line isn't enough—especially if you're targeting something that's unrealistic. If you're a hundred pounds overweight and haven't exercised in years, for instance, is saying that you're going to be a marathon runner in two months realistic? And if it's not realistic, is it going to keep you motivated? Probably not.

That's why I'm such a big fan of finding your *real why*. It encourages you to connect with your life *right now*, find an appropriate starting point, and celebrate your daily victories along the way. Motivation may be fickle, but a *why* you can believe in will help sustain you even on the bad days.

PRACTICAL DOUG

My father-in-law, whom you're going to hear more about throughout this book, was a go-getting, high-achieving professional and public servant throughout his impressive career. He's now seventy, retired, and wants to be as in-charge of his health as ever. He has had some negative interactions with doctors in the past and isn't one to accept a recommendation that he doesn't understand or agree with.

Doug was working two jobs and was not particularly focused on his health when his wife, my mother-in-law, was diagnosed with pancreatic cancer. The hospital that she was being treated at was more than an hour's drive from their house, but only six miles from ours. Plus, I was well-connected at my home institution and would be joining her and Doug for all of her appointments. The practical step was for them to move in with us for as long as she needed to.

On the day they arrived, Doug struggled to carry their bags from their car to their new bedroom. As he did so, he came to an important realization: if he couldn't even carry his wife's suitcases without feeling winded, he was worried he would have difficulty helping take care of her. For someone like Doug, this simply wasn't an option.

His desire to help his wife as she lived with cancer for the next two years became his *real why*. As a high-level professional, Doug was used to having control. While he couldn't control his wife's illness, he *could* control his own body so he could be a better partner on her journey. He wasn't interested in becoming a male swimsuit model or a triathlete. He simply wanted to walk without losing his breath, to carry his wife's bags, and to help her through her many hospital visits without needing to join her as a patient! In these ways, Doug's *real why* connected to his life, was achievable, and didn't involve any complicated diet plans or expensive equipment. Most importantly, however, this strong, intelligent (if somewhat stubborn) man had to come to this decision on his own.

Even as Doug began his health-up journey, I held back from offering advice, knowing he would ask if he wanted it. Mostly, I lived my own healthy habits and unknowingly (at the time) became a good example. He started going for walks. First, it was just around the block. Gradually, he would go farther and farther. His habit grew with each step. As he started banking wins, his confidence and know-how grew.

With people like my father-in-law, the finish line doesn't sustain them. There isn't necessarily a huge end goal like running a marathon. Instead, it's about being healthy for the journey. We don't believe we can get there because the amount of work required scares us. But Doug isn't easily scared and his *why* was strong. What once looked like a mountain became nothing more than a series of small hills.

HOW REAL PEOPLE FIND THEIR *REAL WHYS*

I've found that a person's *real why* is rarely due to abstract medical reasons. Sure, most people understand, for instance, that healthy living dramatically reduces the risk of a heart attack. However, unless they've seen someone actually have a heart attack, the idea usually doesn't resonate. It's too far away from their real-world experience. Sadly, the reality often doesn't strike until they find themselves in the ER with me.

HITTING BOTTOM

Real whys are usually connected to what I call "rough-bottom" moments. These are often accompanied by a trip to the ER with a series of super-scary symptoms like chest pains, blurry vision, and difficulty breathing. This is when abstraction becomes reality.

Some people need to hit those rough-bottom moments before they can get serious about taking care of themselves. For others, seeing it happen to a friend or a loved one is enough. Either way, once you've witnessed or experienced one of these rough-bottom moments, you'll start to see the importance of turning your own life around.

One day, during a typical shift in the ER, a patient arrived who had suffered a heart attack and needed a heart catheterization and stents. I'm not sure why, but that day I was particularly fired up. I wanted to give him the most empowering cheerleading speech I could muster. As we were preparing him for his procedure, he and I had a talk.

"Smoking caused this," I said. "But we were able to catch

it in time, and I don't think you're going to have a lot of damage. I want you to tell yourself that this is the day you get your life back. You had your last cigarette on the way in here today, but no more." Imagine this in a loud, excited voice with lots of hand gestures. I'm passionate at baseline—this was me in turbo mode!

Six months later, the man was back for an unrelated injury. I didn't recognize him at first and was going through my standard questionnaire. When I asked if he had ever been a smoker, he looked at me and said, "Dr. Hope, don't you remember me? I'm the guy you put the fear of God into after my heart attack." Now, while I would love to say I can remember every patient's face that has come through my emergency room, when you're caring for hundreds of new faces in that time, sometimes you need to do a double-take before a former patient registers with you. After taking a moment to let his face register, our past encounter came rushing back, and my eyes lit up.

"Yes, I remember you now!" I said. "How are things going?"

"I quit smoking that day," he said. "I feel great. You helped change my life."

I couldn't help it. I broke into tears and gave him a big hug. However, I wasn't about to let him give me all the credit. "*You* helped change your life," I said. "*You* were the one open to the message. All I did was help give you what you needed."

It was a great moment to follow up with someone, a moment I'm rarely afforded as an ER doctor.

This man's story could have ended a lot differently. He could just as easily have been fatalistic after his heart attack. He could have said, "Well, I'm screwed," and put another cigarette in his mouth. Instead, the rough bottom helped him realize he could choose his own destiny and embrace healthier habits in his life.

The thing about change is that *you* have to change in order to change. Some of my favorite quotes and memes around this are:

"Don't expect a change if you don't make one"

"If you don't change, nothing will change."

"If you want something you've never had, you need to do something you've never done."

My patient had found himself in a moment where he was ready to change. And although the decision was made in a single moment, he still ran into barriers (i.e., cravings) as he stuck with this change. His *why* was stronger than his desire to smoke. He wanted something he didn't have and made it his new habit.

EVERYONE'S *WHY* IS DIFFERENT

Luckily, not everyone needs a heart attack and a fired-up presurgery speech to motivate them. Everyone's *real why* is a little different. Most are personal, expressing hopes, fears, and dreams far too specific for me to suggest to anyone else.

I knew one woman who'd heard that secondhand smoke could give her dog cancer. Forget the damage she was doing to herself—the idea that she could be hurting her pet became her *real why* for quitting.

I knew another woman who said, "That bitch Heather is skinnier than me! I will not live in a world where she is better than me in any way." It certainly wasn't the friendliest of *whys*, but if it got her going every day, then the result is the same.

Your *real why* might be the most empowering idea in the world. It might come as a result of your darkest moment. It might even be an external motivator, like a dog or a rival. Ultimately, it doesn't matter what it is. You don't need to impress anyone with your reason. You just need to have one.

NERD ALERT: WHY YOUR DOCTOR
DOESN'T HELP YOU GET FIT

There's a common complaint that doctors only intervene when a patient's health goes south. They treat the problem, but they rarely help prevent it.

It's a legitimate concern—and a real problem. Let's talk a little bit about why that is.

In med school, aspiring doctors usually spend the first two years learning how the body works and the next two years learning how to treat diseases. Sometimes they learn a little bit about human behavior along the way, but it's rarely a point of focus. Historically, if they wanted to go in-depth about human behavior, they'd have to do it on their own time.

But as we've already discussed, finding time is tricky. Treating patients is a lot of work. Many doctors *want* to spend more time discussing preventative care, but opportunities to do so are rare—and, unfortunately, they're not always incentivized.

Doctors are often reimbursed per procedure rather than by outcome. If they set a bone, perform a surgery, or put in sutures, they get paid. However, if they spend an hour talking to you about health-positive habits, they don't get reimbursed the same way.

It's not that doctors are greedy, but they do need to pay their student loans, pay their employees, and keep the lights in the office on, just like everybody else. Unfortunately, this creates a vacuum. When doctors can't talk to their patients, those patients start looking for answers elsewhere.

That's where unlicensed health gurus and fad diets come in. To be fair, not all unlicensed practitioners are quacks. Some know their stuff and are doing the medical world a complementary service. But there are a lot of charlatans out there trying to sell snake oil to people who don't know any better.

Fortunately, the medical world is changing. Education has begun to prioritize preventative care and human behavior change. Medical reimbursement is shifting toward a more outcome-based model. Some of these shifts may lead to other unintended consequences, but for now, they're a step in the right direction.

OUR FOUR PATIENTS FIND THEIR *REAL WHYS*

Excited about finding your *real why*? Great! Before you move on to the next chapter, let's check in on our four patients to learn about their *real whys*.

SARAH

In a blissful moment of downtime, Sarah is watching her

three daughters play house. The oldest is dutifully performing the role of "mommy," pretending to take care of the younger kids.

But what Sarah hears next stops her dead in her tracks. When the four-year-old asks the seven-year-old "mommy" who takes care of *her*, the latter replies, "Oh no, Mommy doesn't need to take care of herself. She takes care of everybody else. Mommies don't matter themselves."

Sarah feels the whole room sink. *What have I taught her?* she thinks, though she already knows the answer.

Ever since she started having kids, Sarah has been running herself into the ground. She's been ignoring her own needs so she could attend to her daughters' needs. Through every day, every behavior, every interaction, her children have internalized this lesson. If this is the example she's setting, how will her daughters raise their own children?

That's not the future Sarah wants for her daughters. Something has to change. *She* has to change.

BILL

It's another busy day for Bill. He's been feeling pretty run-down lately, but he's the boss and if he doesn't stay on his game, the problems will just keep piling up.

During a particularly high-stakes meeting, Bill is having trouble concentrating. The shortness of breath he's felt before has returned, but this time, it's accompanied by this strange pressure that's affecting his vision, making everything look hazy and light.

Bill can't worry about that now. He has a big deal to land, and he needs to concentrate.

He's able to focus for a few more minutes, but then the nausea kicks in. Unable to ignore it, Bill gets up, excuses himself, and heads to the men's room.

As Bill splashes cold water on his face, he looks up at the mirror and sees his dad. For the first time, Bill realizes he's the same age as his father when he died of a heart attack.

It's not just the physical resemblance, Bill realizes. In every way, he's his father's son. He is the same hard-driving, no-days-off kind of guy, living as if they handed out trophies for the most self-sacrifice.

As the pain in Bill's chest surges, all these thoughts fall away. Struggling to stay on his feet, Bill fumbles for his phone and dials 911.

MARY

There are only so many chores to do in an empty house. The laundry is done, everything is dusted, and Mary can only straighten up the mementos her kids left behind so many times.

In the hallway, Mary stops.

"Who am I?" she says to herself. She's not singularly focused on being John and Susan's mom anymore. She has nothing to do and no one to take care of. What is she going to do with this empty house and all this empty space?

Mary walks to the closet and locates the box of old keepsakes from high school. There's the picture of her with her volleyball team, and the second-place ribbon they won during the state finals. "What could I have been?" Mary asks. But after a moment, she realizes it's not the right question.

Mary is grateful for what has been a wonderful life, and she doesn't regret a moment of it. But standing in the hallway, she realizes how much life she still has left to live. "What *else* can I do?" Mary says, finally breaking the silence. "Who else can I be?"

GEORGE

Recovering from his recent knee surgery, George has begun to catalogue his various aches and pains. In some ways, he considers the pain a good trade-off for a life well lived. He likes the career he had, the friends he made, and the things he accomplished. He's set in his ways, sure, but those ways have always served him well.

However, now that his body has kinks in places he doesn't even have a name for, George is starting to wonder if that upstart newbie who wanted to bring yoga into the shop was right all along. Maybe he wasn't some weirdo hippie after all.

He knows that's not what really bothers him. The aches and pains George can deal with. But his doctor's parting words have really been sticking in his craw. "You're getting by," the doctor said, "but with the shape you're in, you don't have much to look forward to other than your recliner and your favorite TV shows."

Well, screw that guy, George thinks. *What does he know? Who's he to say what I can or can't do?*

WHAT WILL BECOME YOUR *REAL WHY*?

Whenever we accomplish a big goal, we always remember our driving forces for getting there.

I still remember the high school teacher who said I wasn't college material and the instructor in med school who suggested I was only there to meet a husband.[4] They fired up my internal obstinate protester and helped give me the resolve to keep going during all those uncertain moments along the way.

In that regard, we're all a little like George. You tell my toddler to eat his broccoli, and he'll look at it like it's poison. Tell him that he *can't* eat his broccoli, and it's gone before I can blink. Defiance makes for a great *real why*, but it's not the only motivator.

Now it's time to ask, what's *your real why*? I'm committed to helping you find it, and I've got just the exercise to help you get there.

THE 12 REASONS EXERCISE

Another one of my favorite memes comes from the TV show *South Park*. In one episode, there is a gang of Under-

---

4   This probably goes without saying, but his statement couldn't have been further from the truth. I had great grades in school, took part in extracurricular activities, and had a job to boot. Although I had to work hard in calculus, I still did fine! It took me years to realize I wasn't the problem. I excelled in college and got accepted to my first-choice med school on my first try. This teacher was just a special brand of jerk who had no business discouraging an insecure high school student like me. And the sexist med school instructor? This guy was just a 157-year-old dinosaur who didn't understand why women were getting into medicine and not staying home barefoot and pregnant. I'm glad to see these prehistoric attitudes falling into the tar pits where they belong. We've come a long way, baby!

pants Gnomes who have developed a whole business model out of stealing underpants.

The problem is they haven't thought it through very well. They know step one is "steal underpants," and they know step three is "profit," but they don't know step two, which they've underscored on their flowchart with a big question mark.

When considering your own *real why*, it's important that you're not an Underpants Gnome. So far in this chapter, you've learned about step one (the value of finding your *real why*), and you've learned about step three (your *real why* helps you live healthier), but we haven't talked about step two: how to actually find your *real why*.

That's where my 12 Reasons exercise comes in. Don't worry, this exercise isn't about doing a routine of sit-ups and burpees. This is about thinking about your reasons for wanting to change—your *whys*.

WHY 12 REASONS?

We rarely tell people our real motivations. Part of that is we're too embarrassed. Another part is we haven't actually thought it through ourselves. This exercise will help you cut through the superficial stuff and find those real reasons.

Say there's a guy who just bought a new Lamborghini. He can talk up the gas mileage and safety features all he wants, but everyone knows he bought it because it makes him feel like a hot piece of ass. The safety features and gas mileage are his first couple reasons—they're logical, but they're also superficial. As he gets further along on his list, however, he starts to make more emotional connections—it looks cool, it makes fun sounds, and he feels good driving it. With one more answer to go, he might actually cop to the hot-piece-of-ass factor.

Just like the Lamborghini driver, whether we admit it or not, most of us make emotional choices rather than logical ones. The logic comes after, and it's usually just a way for us to justify our emotional choices. When you do the 12 Reasons exercise, your first few reasons for getting healthy will sound incredibly logical—losing a few pounds puts less strain on your joints, quitting smoking helps prevent lung cancer, eight hours of rest reduces the risk of heart disease, and so on and so forth.

These are good reasons, but they're probably not your *real* reasons. I want you to get to the good stuff. I want you to tap that raw emotion. I want you to recognize what *really* drives you.

In my experience, it's going to take listing several reasons to get there.

WHAT DO YOU WANT—OR WANT TO AVOID?

For some, the 12 Reasons exercise leads them to a specific goal. A mother once admitted to me that she wanted to be able to walk her kids to the park without losing her breath. Another woman confided that for the first time in her adult life, she wanted to feel comfortable having sex with the lights on and no T-shirt to cover her.

For others, the 12 Reasons exercise led them to outcomes they wanted to avoid. One man didn't want to have a heart attack at forty-five like all the other men in his family. One woman wanted to quit smoking because she didn't want to get wrinkles. A younger student I worked with wanted to avoid another embarrassing moment where she got stuck in her seat during an assembly.

Whatever your *real why* is, know that you're valid at any size and in any state. It's okay to love yourself no matter where you are with your goals. Part of this exercise is about allowing yourself to be uncomfortable, but the other part is about loving yourself enough to believe that getting where you want to be is possible.

READY TO START?

Now that I've explained the exercise, here's what I want you to do.

First, stop reading and go find a pencil. Next, start writing. Whether you write in your book or on a separate piece of paper, I want you to do this *for real*. This is a workbook, and the 12 Reasons exercise is your homework.

You don't start living healthier through osmosis. This is your chance to change—and to find your reason for doing so.

At a conference, I was listening to a keynote by Jesse Itzler, author of *Living with a SEAL: 31 Days Training with the Toughest Man on the Planet*. He recalled a moment when he and his kid were playing with the hose in their yard. As the fun wound down, Itzler started to walk away, telling himself that he'd put the hose away later. Then he stopped. "How you do something is how you do everything," he said, remembering an old saying from someone he admired, and then he walked back over and put the hose away.

With the 12 Reasons exercise, here's your chance to live up to those words. How you move forward now is how you're going to move forward with each habit from here on out. So take a moment to do it right. Remember, though, that while I recommend writing out a full twelve reasons, I don't recommend simply picking the twelfth by default. Pick the one that resonates, that makes you feel self-conscious, that you would hide from others if you were writing this down in public.

When you're done, come meet me in Chapter 2.

CHAPTER 2

OBSTACLES AND MOTIVATION

How did you like that last chapter? Did it make you feel motivated, like you can take on anything? It did? Great!

Admit it, though: part of your brain is thinking, *Oh no! I can't ever have a doughnut again.*

Yep, I can read your mind. I know all about those pesky objections that creep in after the initial surge of motivation.

Fear not, however. It's natural to feel some chatter and pushback from your brain. Maybe you're thinking about how much time and money your new Habit That lifestyle is going to take. Maybe you're thinking that it conflicts with your current lifestyle. Maybe you're still thinking about those doughnuts.

It's okay if you are. I'm not judging.

However, rather than let obstacles become objections that derail your hard work, in this chapter, you're going to learn how to recognize these roadblocks and steer around them.

OBSTACLES ARE A GOOD THING

"The difference between an obstacle and an adventure is your attitude."

Who doesn't love a sense of accomplishment? When you're an infant, it's all about taking your first steps. A few years later, it's all about learning to run and ride a bike. And a little bit after that, if you're my kids anyway, it's all about tumbling, flipping, and leaping through an obstacle course your mommy took a half hour to build.

I like obstacles. Without them, I'd never feel like I accomplished anything. Do you know how good it's felt being able to keep at this book even though I've been recovering from appendicitis and working two jobs? Take *that*, life!

Obstacles are part of the human experience. But as the

following stories show, there are plenty of ways to make them work *for* us rather than let them stand in our way.

MY FRIEND MEETS THE GIRL OF HIS DREAMS

Some years ago, a friend of mine was at a bar with buddies, talking to girls and feeling confident and sassy, when he looked up at a balcony and saw a woman. As he described it to me, the very sight of her made his heart leap, so he motioned at her to come down.

She looked at him, shook her head, and motioned for him to come up instead. He told me he's never flown up a flight of stairs faster in his life. The place was completely packed, but it was as if he grew wings and flew up to that balcony completely unimpeded.

He is now happily married to the balcony babe.

MY KIDS VERSUS THE OBSTACLE COURSE

As I said, a while back my kids begged me to set up the house like a big obstacle course. I made one. I worked really hard on it, and when it was done, they tore right through it in no time flat.

The second they were done, they loved it so much they demanded another one. I gave them a new challenge instead. "Do it again," I said, "but this time hopping on one foot—and the floor is lava!"

Off they went on another adventure.

MY FATHER-IN-LAW GOES FOR A WALK

You already met my father-in-law in Chapter 1. He's a wonderful, smart man who doesn't like being told what to do. Back in the day when he was Douglas Roberts, Treasurer for the State of Michigan, he would go to the doctor's office and then choose what he would allow to be done. Certain blood tests were okay, but not others. *He* was in the driver's seat, and *he* was going to choose based on his values.

Doug takes orders from no one, so his *real why* was never going to come from anyone besides himself. After he came to live with us for a while, he saw me living the Habit That life—saw how easy it was—and said, "Oh, I can do that too."

When he was ready, and *only* on his own terms, he decided he was going to go for a walk.

WHAT'S THE POINT?

Each of the people in these stories had obstacles, but they

also had specific goals they were trying to reach. When you want something badly enough, all the obstacles melt away.

However, as we're about to find out, the opposite is true as well. If you *don't* want something badly, you'll have no problem finding an obstacle and hiding behind it. A tiny housefly can seem like a formidable fire-breathing dragon when the effort it takes to conquer it is more than the will you have for the task—though, spoiler alert, the opposite is true as well. Trust me, you can try just about anything without bursting into flames (unless you're literally playing with fire, of course). In the rest of this chapter, you're going to learn how to get there.

THE OBSTACLE/OBJECTION RELATIONSHIP

Before we go any further, I do want to be clear on one point: obstacles are real. I didn't invent the appendicitis that interrupted my writing of this book, nor my mother-in-law's cancer. I'm sure your life is also full of very real things standing in the way of the healthy habits you want to build.

Even with two kids, two jobs, speaking gigs, a social circle that means the world to me, and that pesky emergency surgery, however, I still wrote this book. If you want the Habit That lifestyle, you'll find a way to get there. The trick is to not let obstacles become objections.

ANYTHING CAN BECOME AN OBSTACLE

There's a joke I like to tell during lectures. First, I'll say that if I want to get my ten thousand steps in, I can walk back and forth across the front of the room as I teach. I get going with my pacing, and then suddenly I drop my book on the floor.

"Oh no, the book is in the way," I say. "I guess that means I can't walk around it. I'll just have to sit instead. And you know what? Now that I'm sitting, I might as well grab a doughnut!"

Naturally, that's ridiculous. The book isn't a real obstacle. However, it's a great way to demonstrate a common human trait. If you don't want to do something badly enough, you're going to hide behind the tiniest excuse not to do it.

That's why finding your *real why* in Chapter 1 is so important. Without it, you'll look for reasons to quit rather than keep going. So if you haven't done that 12 Reasons exercise yet, I suggest you flip back to it and get cracking.

SAYING IT OUT LOUD MAKES IT REAL

Here's another truth of human nature. If you say something, you believe it.

It happens to everyone, even to toddlers. Once we've said

something out loud, we'll dig in and argue our position until we're blue in the face. Political debates on Facebook are a perfect example. Each party starts with a preconceived opinion of what's true and not true, right and wrong, and tries vainly to convince the other. As the argument progresses, each participant (likely there are more than two by now) digs their heels in deeper until, in a sad twist of psychology, they actually believe their side even *more* than they had before the argument started! (If you're like me, though, you have no interest in such threads and instead wander away to hilarious memes and funny animal videos.)

This is important to keep in mind on those days you're not feeling it (and more on that in just a second). Sure, you could say, "I'm out," and be done with it. But here's a question: What would you say to your best friend if they were feeling similarly beat down? Would you tell them to quit, or would you tell them to get back on that horse and give at least five minutes to building good habits?

Now ask yourself, "*If that's what I would tell my best friend, why would I tell myself any different?*"

WHAT ABOUT THE BAD DAYS?

One of my favorite thought leaders, Genius Network founder Joe Polish, said, "The difference between the amateurs and the professionals is that the professionals do it with a headache." Theodore Roosevelt once said, "Nothing worth having was ever achieved without effort." And he would know. He once delivered a speech *after* getting shot in the chest!

Not every day is going to be perfect. If you came into this book expecting me to tell you otherwise, you're about to be disappointed.

On the bad days, remember these two things:

#1. The Feeling Follows the Action

If you're waiting for that perfect burst of motivation, you are never going to reach your goals. You'll find an obstacle, then you'll find an objection, and then you'll find the couch.

The feeling follows the action, not the other way around. I can't tell you how many times I didn't feel like working out, did it anyway, and felt incredible afterward. I'm sure you've experienced the same thing. Go out and find that feeling!

#2. Be Human

We often think that healthy living means we have to be

on all the time, that we have to be happy, sunny people like the health gurus we see on TV. We say, "Oh, I'm supposed to be this amazing, perfect, healthy-habits person 24/7 and levitate on a cloud of constant awesomeness and bliss." The truth is, even the gurus are real people and have bad days. They simply have more practice staying on track during the inevitable ups and downs of life.

For us "mere mortals," the whole process of motivating ourselves to be motivated is both exhausting and unnecessary. We put that on ourselves. No one else expects that of us.

Keep these two things in mind for those days that are just ridiculous and shitty. On my nineteenth birthday, I was riding my bike to class and got hit by a car. I was scraped up and pretty indignant (after all, I had the right of way, given that I was on the sidewalk!). Fortunately, I suffered no permanent injuries and wound up being fine, although my bike was totaled. If that wasn't disheartening enough, later that day, I ended up in the ER with food poisoning! To this day, the smell of lemon chicken soup still evokes a nausea response (ugh!).

It's okay to suck at life on days like that. You can't be super motivated every single day. On that crap day, I didn't care about the burpees and broccoli. I just wanted a hug and a nap! Don't beat yourself up over your own crap days. If you can, try to grab five healthy minutes to health up. If you can't, just remind yourself that you're going to try for a little more the next day.

WHAT IF THE OBJECTIONS LURE YOU BACK IN?

I'd love to think that reading this chapter is going to be all it takes for you to overcome your objections once and for all. The truth is, you may return to your objections regardless of my advice. If you believe them enough, it doesn't matter what I say. It's up to you to find a way forward.

When that happens, the Habit That Tribe and I would love to hear from you. Go to Facebook, find our group (again, that's "The Habit That Tribe"[5]), and tell us your biggest objections and how you can get over them. Then, I want you to take that exercise one step further and help someone else who's struggling to learn how to crush their own objections.

As my mom has reminded me more than once, "Sometimes courage is just a quiet voice reminding you to try again tomorrow." Here's your chance to be that voice for someone else.

---

5   https://www.facebook.com/groups/1983040705045797/

COMMON OBJECTIONS TO BUILDING HEALTHY HABITS

In the next section, I'm going to systematically destroy the most common healthy living objections I hear. Maybe you've used one or more of these objections, or maybe your objection is something else entirely. Either way, these will help you get a better sense of how to recognize when you're standing in your own way, and what to do about it.

OBJECTION #1: I DON'T KNOW HOW TO APPLY ALL THE KNOWLEDGE

If there's a gap in your knowledge, it's hard to feel empowered to make healthy choices. What if you don't know how to use this squat press machine? What if you don't know how to prepare healthy meals?

These are legitimate concerns, so high-five yourself for recognizing that. The good news is that most knowledge gaps are easily fixable, and if you commit to making a habit out of learning, you may even find the process empowering.

In other words, instead of giving up on the gym because you don't know how to use the squat machine, keep your promise. Go to the gym and either find something that you *do* understand or commit to learning something new.

Good Intentions, Bad Information

"Did you know that shoving two sticks of unsalted butter and a pickle up your ass cures cancer? You can trust me: I am a random picture on Facebook."

Here's the million-dollar question: if you're going to learn, where should you get your information?

This question is especially relevant when it comes to our food choices. You've probably noticed how much conflicting diet advice is out there. One camp tells you to eat nothing but bacon. Another tells you it's all about the carbs. Yet another camp comes out of left field and says eggs are the best food ever. The next day, a fourth camp swoops in and says eggs are the worst and that you will probably burst into flames if you're even in the same room with them.

All this advice sounds reasonably legit, and some of it even comes from doctors. So whom do you trust?

Part of building healthy habits is learning to be a filter. When you're out there Googling healthy information, try this. First, recognize your biases. Second, focus on *quality* rather than quantity.

This means knowing how to recognize credible sources. The health advice you receive should be:

1. Free from the influence of lobbying groups or other interests
2. Based on provable scientific fact
3. Produced by credible organizations with dedicated professionals in their field
4. Personally, I like the Mayo Clinic, the University of Michigan, and NutritionFacts.org, run by Dr. Michael Greger. They're great at providing the big picture and combining their recommendations with sound scientific reasoning.
5. Wherever you get your information, especially when it comes to diet and weight loss, remember that there are lots of fad diets and memes out there. Seriously, I saw a meme one time that suggested sticking a buttered pickle up your butt to fight cancer—which, I'm sorry to report, does not work. If your goal is only to lose weight, any one of those fads will probably work in the short term, but they won't be very helpful in building lifelong healthy habits.

It's Okay If You Feel Overwhelmed

With conflicting information—and changing information—it's easy to feel overwhelmed. But don't let that feeling of being overwhelmed become a cop-out.

In the next chapter, you'll learn how to break your goals down into small actions. Crafting a perfect diet or the perfect workout may sound tough, but I bet drinking more water or eating one green vegetable every day sounds much more manageable. Remember, healthing up involves one five-minute change at a time. No need to overwhelm yourself and quit. I'd rather you do something small than nothing at all.

Learning takes time, so just remember that you don't have to take care of it all at once. Do what you can today, then do a little more tomorrow.

OBJECTION #2: WHY BOTHER TRYING? I'VE ALREADY TRIED A MILLION THINGS

Sometimes I catch myself watching late-night infomercials like some people watch horror movies. "No, don't buy that!" I scream at the TV, hoping somehow other viewers will hear me and not spend their hard-earned money on strange, complicated, and too-good-to-be-true contraptions. Sadly, they never do.

The weight loss industry is a roughly $40-billion-a-year industry. It's safe to say most of us have spent some money on a fitness gadget or two. I hate to break it to you, but that two hundred bucks you spend on the vibrating ab belt probably isn't going to do your midsection much good.

I sympathize if the myriad things you've tried haven't

panned out. However, the question is, how legitimate were those diets and devices, and how long did you try them?

Any day you eat healthy is a great day. However, if you only ate superhealthy for three days and were disappointed you didn't lose fifty pounds, that's unrealistic. By all means, keep at the healthy eating habits. The weight *will* come off—don't give up! However, in order to feel successful, you have to make sure your goals align with reality.

It's also important to remember that diet and exercise are just two of our four pillars. If you're sleep-deprived and stressed out, there may be other reasons you're not seeing the results you want.

OBJECTION #3: I'M DOING EVERYTHING RIGHT AND I'M STILL NOT SEEING CHANGES

One time, during a talk I was giving on the value of healthy eating, a gentleman in the audience kept objecting to my message.

"Eating healthy food makes you fatter," he said. "Doing everything right makes you gain weight."

I wanted to say, "Dude, that is not how you science," but I

let it go and found him afterward. As we spoke, I learned that he drank two gallons of whole milk a day. Two full gallons! Because he'd learned as a kid that "milk does a body good," he figured the more he drank, the better—never mind how many calories he was taking in.

I was glad I understood his objections better. He had good intentions, but he was a little misguided. More than anything, however, I was impressed. That's *a lot* of milk to drink every day.

Check Your Assumptions

You've probably noticed there's a lot of misinformation out there when it comes to healthy habits. Competing with actual science is a lot of lobbying and marketing. Some of the hokey stuff we can spot, but some of it's ingrained in us from a young age.

Just like living the Habit That life takes time, so does getting all your facts straight. Check your assumptions and try to learn more where you can. Just because milk is marketed as a healthy food doesn't mean your body is going to respond well to a calorie overload.

Are You Really Counting Every Calorie?

Speaking of calories, I've worked with plenty of people

who are genuinely trying. They show me their food diaries, and I can see for myself that they really are eating well.

At least, they're making good choices with the foods they remember to write down. The problem is, it's easy to forget to write down what we call *insensible calories*.

If you've ever been a calorie counter, perhaps this sounds familiar. You wrote down your breakfast and kept track of your lunch—but somehow that bowl of M&M's you were grazing on at your coworker's desk didn't make it into your journal!

Whether or not you remember to write those calories down, your body counts them just the same. Those little snacking moments may not sound like much, but they can add up if you're not factoring them in.

OBJECTION #4: I DON'T HAVE THE TIME OR MONEY FOR THIS

Not to sound too much like an old-timer, but back in the day, if you wanted to listen to a song, you had to wait until it came on the radio, or at least until you could fast-forward your cassette tape to the right spot. Now, when my kids want to go retro and hear *The Lion King* soundtrack, they get impatient when I take too long downloading it from the cloud.

Modern life has trained us to expect instant results. Unfortunately, this attitude doesn't work too well when it comes to our bodies.

No Time, Lots of Money

I was working in wellness at a side job when a patient came in for a liposuction consult. She was an executive at a high-stress job. She didn't have much spare time, but she sure had a lot of money.

My job was to consult with her on the benefits of a healthy lifestyle, but she was having none of it. "Where is the surgeon?" she said. "I want to eat whatever I want. And then I'm going to come in here every year or two and get it all liposuctioned off."

My jaw fell to the floor. I tried to explain to her that wasn't how liposuction works. Our bodies have two kinds of fat: (1) the subcutaneous (under the skin) kind that sits outside of our muscles that we can suck out, and (2) the visceral fat inside the abdominal cavity around our organs that lipo can't get to. The only way to get rid of the visceral fat, I explained, was through diet and exercise.

It took two different doctors to convince her there was nothing we could do. Despite our efforts, she still stormed off, indignant, and likely went elsewhere to see if less reputable doctors would be willing to help her.

Because you picked up this book, I know you're not that kind of person. You've read this far because you understand that building healthy habits takes time and there's no such thing as a quick fix when it comes to our bodies. And the good news is, because you put in the work, you're going to feel a hell of a lot better than the misguided lipo lady.

I Don't Want to Wait!

"Never give up on a dream because of the time it will take to accomplish it. The time will pass anyway."

People don't like to hear that losing weight takes time. But the way I see it, the year is going to pass anyway. How do you want it to go?

No matter what, you're going to be accomplishing some remarkable stuff throughout the year. So why not create some new healthy habits and make that one of your accomplishments?

Nothing else in life happens immediately. You don't make partner at a law firm by the second week. Similarly, you don't gain all the weight you don't want overnight—and you can't lose it overnight either.

We're all waiting for this magical utopian moment where we have all this free time. But for 99 percent of us, our calendar is never going to magically open up.

We're all busy. I have two kids, two dogs, and two jobs. (By my reckoning, I think that means I deserve two husbands.) Many of my patients have a lot more going on than I do.

At certain times in my life, I've had two or three hours a day of free time to work with. At other points, I was lucky to have fifteen minutes. In either case, I did what I could and didn't beat myself up over what I couldn't.

If guilt and self-loathing burned calories, we would all be skinny. But it doesn't. So let's be realistic instead.

What About Time for Family?

I'm all about healthy habits, but I'm not about sacrificing family. Just remember that it doesn't have to be an either/or. If you work out *with* your kids, you're spending quality time while teaching your kids to be fit and have fun. Plus, having family gives you built-in workout partners. Keeping up with my maniac kids and two big dogs has given me plenty of exercise!

Isn't Eating Organic Expensive?

From my experience, the idea that organic food is more expensive is somewhat of a myth. But you don't have to eat organic to eat healthy. Traditionally, farmed broccoli is still better for you than a doughnut.

Don't forget to factor in the costs of *not* eating healthy as well. Sure, the junk food you're eating now may be cheaper in the checkout lane than the organic broccoli, but the long-term health costs and the missed time from work aren't.

Eating any vegetable is better than no vegetable. I'll leave the details to you, but otherwise, my suggestion is to decide on something you want to eat and apply the money.

Gyms Are Expensive, Too

It's true. A lot of gyms aren't cheap. But you know what is? YouTube. Not only is it free, but it's like having a personal trainer in your room!

Just like you don't have to buy organic, free-range, grass-fed, frequently massaged beef to be healthier, you don't need a gym membership. You can squat for free. You can jog up and down the street for free. You can do burpees for free. You can run up and down the stairs in most buildings for free (although try not to get security called on you).

OBJECTION #5: NOW IS NOT A GOOD TIME

When I'm teaching medical students, I tell them I'm not there to teach them how to teach their patients how to live better. I'm there to teach *my students* how to live better.

After giving them a moment to nod along, I keep going. "But of course, you're busy med students," I say. "You have a ton of exams coming up that you've got to study for. So really, your first couple years of med school aren't a good time because you're super busy in bookwork. You can wait until the third year.

"Oh, wait, no," I continue. "By then, you're going to be doing all your clinical work and spending all your time in hospitals, so that's not a good time. And same with residency, I guess. That'll be super busy, and you're going to be working a ton of hours, so that's not a great time either."

This goes on for a while, with me painstakingly describing how every point in their lives will be endlessly busy until I'm certain that everybody in the room gets the point.

If you keep waiting for the right time, you're going to be retired one day, like George, wondering if now it's too late.

Sometimes people protest that healthy habits are impossible if they want to eat out at restaurants or enjoy the holidays.

I really, really want you to enjoy restaurants and holidays. I'm not asking you to cut out fun. The Habit That lifestyle wouldn't be worth very much to anyone if it wasn't any fun. My goal is to help you integrate healthier habits into who you are *right now*, not to cut out all the things you love for the rest of time.

OBJECTION #6: IT JUST DOESN'T FIT WHO I AM

Identity is a crazy thing. If you don't see yourself as a healthy person, or if you think healthy habits somehow interfere with the kind of person you want to be, then you risk letting this kind of objection become a real obstacle. Here are three of the most common identity objections I tend to see.

#1. The Rebel

While giving a volunteer motivational talk at a local community center, I met a kid in his early twenties. He was a rebel. "I don't eat that healthy crap because no one's going to tell me what to do," he told me.

That was who he was, and I told him I thought it was awesome. Then I said, "You know what? If you use that spirit for good instead of evil, you'll probably change the world."

Everyone laughed, but the most important thing is that the kid was right. He *was* being told what to do—just not by me. I just wanted him to feel good and live the life he wanted.

The truth is, most of us are exposed to thousands of marketing messages each day. Marketers have long known that equating unhealthy products with freedom and rebelliousness is good business. They train us to think the only way we can be real rebels is by buying their junk food or smoking their cigarettes. The reality is we're playing right into their hands.

I assured the kid that Big Broccoli wasn't manipulating him. They didn't have the budget. However, much larger interests *did* have the budget, and they were more than happy to use it. If he really wanted to be a rebel, I said, he'd stop listening to these phony marketing messages and start finding out on his own what was for real.

#2. The Fat Kid

I grew up with someone who was skinny and scrawny as a kid, but gained weight as he moved through his teenage years into adulthood. Eventually, he started calling himself "the fat kid" as a joke, jiggling his belly and saying, "Bring on the bacon!" for emphasis. The longer he did this, the more he really incorporated it into his identity.

In reality, he wasn't *that* overweight, but more and more, he ate and behaved like the fat kid he said he was. If I asked if he wanted to go for a bike ride, he'd reply, "Nope, I'm the fat kid."

Eventually, I got angry, and one day I called him on it. "You will never refer to yourself as the fat kid in front of me again," I said. "You need to let go of that label."

He's still working on the labels he gives himself, but he's not alone. A lot of us struggle with this. We believe the things we call ourselves, but the good news is we can use that power for good, too. For instance, I didn't have the nerve to write this book until I started calling myself a badass author.

#3. The Macho Man

A lot of patients and people I know think healthy equals hippie. That doesn't feel authentic to a lot of people, so they avoid making health-forward decisions because of how it might look.

I get it. I'm a big believer in looking after my mental health, but I couldn't get my brain still to practice meditation if my life depended on it. Despite my aversion to mind-clearing meditation, however, I see myself as a healthy person—and a healthy person takes care of all four pillars.

So how do I take mental breaks in a way that's authentic for me? I go for walks. I like to be in motion, I like being outside and seeing the trees, and I've found this practice allows me to focus, think my best thoughts, and relax.

We'll get into more detail about stress release strategies in Chapter 7, but the point is, you can find healthy habits that are authentically you. If something doesn't feel authentic, don't give up on being a healthy person. Just don't do the things that bother you, and find an alternative that you enjoy.

WHAT DO YOU BELIEVE ABOUT YOURSELF?

At Verne Harnish's ScaleUp Summit, speaker Ari Weinzweig, founder of Zingermans, led the audience through what he called the "This I Believe" exercise. The instructions were straightforward. He gave us a prompt, and then we wrote down the things we believed about ourselves.

For instance, one prompt was, "If people want to hang out with you, what do you believe about yourself?" I found myself writing down all sorts of revealing things. For instance, "Maybe people don't really want to hang out with me because I'm a dork."

Then he asked us to challenge these assumptions. Was I *really* a dork? If so, why do I have all the friends I have—and why do they call and ask to hang out? Why did so many of them bring me flowers, little gifts, and lovingly homemade food when I had my appendix out?

I was grateful to this process for helping me challenge my inner vision of myself. Afterward, I was ready to drop the dork label once and for all, but I knew I had to replace it with something else. So, I decided I'm not a dork, but I *am* a healthy person. I *am* an athlete. I *am* fun to be around because so many things excite me. I am also a science nerd—a label that I proudly embrace.

Take a moment to challenge some of your own labels for yourself. What words come to mind? Are you clumsy? Are you lazy? Are you a total quitter/loser who can never stick to anything because you never have before? List all those negative labels, and then take a good, long look at the things you're calling yourself.

Now, write out the areas in your life where you're success-ful. Maybe you kick ass at your job. Maybe you've surprised even yourself at how good you are at raising a family. Maybe you're an unstoppable force on trivia nights.

The point is, if you're reading this book as the fat kid, you're going to do a fat-kid job with it. But if you read this book as a healthy person, you're going to get a lot more out of it.

OUR PATIENTS' OBJECTIONS

Now that you've learned all about the many types of obstacles to motivation and how you can overcome them, let's take a look at our patients and see what their objections might be.

SARAH

When we last saw Sarah, she was enjoying a bit of downtime watching her kids play. Suddenly, one of her daughters said, "Oh no, Mommy doesn't need to take care of herself. She takes care of everybody else. Mommies don't matter themselves."

Hearing something like that is a punch in the gut. But Sarah realized that's exactly what she'd been teaching her kids. Wearing that mom label, she constantly put herself last. Her kids got first dibs at everything—clothes, love, time, resources, food, you name it.

Sarah wants to change, but those pesky objections keep getting in the way. Between her job and her family, she barely has a waking moment to herself. Besides, spending money on finding a solution means not being able to put food on the table for her kids.

She feels stuck, but she's about to learn just how much small changes can impact her day-to-day reality.

BILL

After excusing himself from a big board meeting, Bill found himself in the bathroom with blurred vision, chest pressure, and a ton of nausea. Just before he collapsed on the floor, he managed to dial 911 and get help.

At the ER, Bill hears his worst fears confirmed: he's had a heart attack. Fortunately, the doctors tell him this wasn't "the Big One." However, if he doesn't start taking care of himself, the Big One is right around the corner.

Bill hears what they're saying, but he's still having trouble admitting he has a problem. After all, he's Superman. He built his business from the ground up through sheer willpower—and dammit, sheer willpower should be able to get him out of this mess, too.

No doubt about it, Bill is fighting against his own pride. He doesn't like being told what to do. He especially doesn't want clients or employees seeing him as weak. But if he can accept that his own choices got him to this point, he'll start to realize that his own choices can get him out of it, too, and actually improve his relationships and effectiveness in the process.

MARY

When Mary came upon those pictures of her old volleyball team, it stopped her dead in her tracks. The so-called glory days may be in the past, but Mary still sees a long road ahead of her. What's next? Who can she be the rest of her life? What can she accomplish?

Mary swells with excitement projecting her life into the future, but a lifetime of false starts continues to hold her back. She's tried the no-carb diet and the cabbage soup diet. She's bought the vibrating ab belts, the dietary supplements, and the hypnosis program. Mary has been there, done that—and none of it worked.

In the back of her mind, Mary knows it's not the products that are the problem. It's her. She never saw herself as a healthy person, but rather as a broken person desperate for a miracle fix. If she can learn to ditch the trendy diets and products and start working on her perspective, though, a big, exciting new world awaits her.

GEORGE

After his knee surgery, George tries to tell himself he's comfortable watching *Matlock* in his favorite recliner. But his doctor's words keep haunting him. The surgery had been a success, but the doctor said his other knee might be next—and then his hips. "With all the stress you're putting on your body, you might as well get used to being in that recliner."

"Screw that guy!" George mumbles to himself. Then, a little louder, "Who says I can't do something?"

Reverse psychology works on some people. It certainly worked here on George. Give up, the doctor says? Hell no. George is a hard worker. He's worked through sick days. He's overcome other injuries. He's *proud* of what he's overcome, and suddenly he's motivated to overcome something else.

George is fully prepared to show that doctor what's what, but then he remembers his knee.

The human knee absorbs up to twenty times a person's body weight with each step. Every extra pound George gains takes him one step further away from recovery. He's afraid to start moving around more, though he knows he'll never feel better unless he does.

"Maybe this is a bad time for me," George says. After all, if he can't go jogging, what can he do realistically anyway?

More and more objections start to creep into George's head. But just as he's about to give in to them, he fights back. "No!" he says. "I want this. I want my life back."

CHAPTER 3

WORK SMARTER, NOT HARDER

Writer Antoine de Saint-Exupéry once said, "A goal without a plan is just a wish." We think we are making goals, but what we are really doing is making a lot of wishes when it comes to our health goals—and a lot of vague wishes at that!

You ever wonder why it's so hard to keep to your weight loss goals, but so easy to head down to your local taco truck? Simply put, "I wanna lose weight" is a vague, abstract concept. Tacos are real and super delicious.

But I'm also a healthy person. And healthy people can still eat tacos and not sweat it. Instead of shaming myself for eating a delicious street taco, I let myself enjoy it. I have my moment. Then, I get on with my healthy life—and find tacos with healthier ingredients.

This chapter is all about learning how to set specific, attainable goals, goals that are as real, fresh, and enticing as your favorite tacos. To get started, let's take a look at a real-world example of what goal setting ends up looking like in our lives.

THE "FAT LADIES' CLUB"

My grandma is in a weight loss group that she lovingly and jokingly calls her "Fat Ladies' Club." This isn't what I would call them; I would never say anything to make such a charming group of people think less of themselves. Besides, it's not even accurate, since the group has several men.[6] That's the image she and her cohorts have going into this, though. It may not be the most proactive mindset, as we talked about last chapter, but, hey, I applaud their desire to live healthier lives.

I've had the privilege of attending this group several times as a guest speaker, and here is what I've observed. At the beginning of every meeting, they have a weigh-in. To make it look like they've done their work, my grandma

---

6   Each of these men, I might add, is just as dedicated to their own health and well-being as any of those ladies. To those men: my grandma may have overlooked you, but I haven't. Way to be proactive with your health!

and some of the other ladies won't eat anything the day of the meeting. Forget that all they're really doing is slowing their metabolism and making long-term weight loss harder. If it takes them a few notches down on the scale, they're all for it!

After the meeting, they're starving, since they haven't eaten much all day. So, they all go out to a restaurant and give themselves permission to eat whatever they want. In a lot of ways, they're as much a social club as a weight loss group, but their intentions are good. To be sure, plenty of the ladies in this group *have* lost weight, but for some, I see habits of deprivation rather than of empowerment.

Sometimes I work with these ladies to help with their goal setting. When I do, I always shoot for interactive conversations, since the best way to get people to set—and stick to—their goals is to have them set those goals themselves. After all, the moment you verbalize something is the moment you start believing it. (If you don't believe me, just watch what happens to a child once they say, "I hate green beans!" I said that twenty-plus years ago, and I'm still sticking to it!)

Besides, it turns out that me wanting something for someone doesn't make *them* want it. As much as I'd love nothing more than to assign health-up practices to everyone, I have learned, sometimes the hard way, that people have to choose their own goals. Otherwise, their goals won't resonate, and they won't stick with them. Even with a Habit That lifer like me, if someone else assigned me to eat green beans, I probably wouldn't stick with it. Yes, I may eat every other veggie under the sun, but that child in my head who said she hated green beans all those years ago still won't let me give them a fair shake...they are icky.

What I've learned from the sessions with my grandma's group is that people are remarkably detailed when relating how they fell off the healthy living wagon. If you ask them what they can do to try and get back on that wagon, it's usually followed by another half-hour of detailed excuses listing all the reasons they can't.

However, when it comes to committing, all the specifics and great storytelling disappear. They simply toss up their hands and make some vague commitment to doing better. They'll start tomorrow, next week, Monday, New Year's Day. The question is, *what* exactly will they start, and *how* do they plan on going about doing it?

Vague plans never resonate. That's why they don't stick. You make yourself a sorta-promise, and then when you fail to follow through on your already shaky commitment, the guilt starts to take over. It all becomes this kind of negative, self-fulfilling prophecy.

For far too many of us, that's what goal-setting looks like. Clearly, it's not that effective, so let's see if we can't hack the system and come up with a better way.

SMARTER GOALS

As I've already said, if losing weight is one of your primary goals, you can follow just about any gimmicky practices and see some short-term results. However, the Habit That way is all about long-term gains by focusing on the goal of becoming a healthy person. If you create healthy habits, the weight loss *will* follow, but that's just a positive symptom of overall good behavior.

That's why I'm a fan of the SMARTER Goals system. Most likely, you've seen this acronym before, or at least variations of it. Usually, the S stands for something like *specific*, just as it does here, while the meaning of the other letters tends to shift around a bit. For our purposes, the SMARTER acronym stands for **S**pecific goals, **M**otivation, **A**ction plan, **R**oadblocks, **T**imetable, **E**volve and evaluate, and **R**ecord and reward.

This chapter will teach you how to use this system and live the Habit That life. At the end, you'll see an example of a SMARTER Goals worksheet, along with a link to download your own and start goal setting. But first, let's talk about each of these elements point-by-point and learn

why they're going to empower you to become a better
goal setter.

STEP 1: SPECIFIC GOALS

In the broadest terms possible, your goal is to be healthier.
Write that at the top of your goals page. It's a great goal,
but it's not very specific. *How* do you want to be healthier?
What does that involve?

Perhaps you want to lose weight. That's a step in the right
direction, but it's still not very specific. Sure, you could
put a more concrete figure on the goal and say, "I want to
lose twenty pounds," but that's still more of an overarch-
ing goal. It's a result, not a plan. It's not effective because
it's not repeatable.

Repetition is the key to learning. Seriously, repetition
is the key to learning (see what I did there?). You don't
learn a tennis serve by practicing it once. You learn it by
practicing it thousands of times. Your SMARTER Goals
will follow this principle. "I want to lose twenty pounds"
may not be a repeatable goal, but eating seven servings
of fruits and vegetables every day *is*. By listing this as one
of your goals, you've given yourself something you can
practice and track every day.

To see other examples of how to create specific goals, visit www.drhopehealth.com. There, you'll find sample action plans for a variety of big-picture goals—whether they're related to diet, exercise, sleep, or stress release.

Sarah Gets Right to the Point

In order to get herself exercising, Sarah knew she had to get as granular as possible with her objectives. The top of her SMARTER Goals worksheet looks something like this:

Be a healthy person.

Get more exercise.

Have more energy and feel less stressed.

Show my children the importance of self-care.

Exercise three times a week for thirty minutes with my kids.

From the big picture (get more exercise) to the specific goal (exercise three times a week with my kids), Sarah's goals feel real. More importantly, they feel *possible*, which allows her to connect with her *why* and stay on track.

But Sarah's taking things a step further. She wants to make sure she actually sees this through. First, she creates an alternative sub-goal: "If I can't exercise for thirty minutes, I can do two fifteen-minute blocks." She also wants to make these specific goals physical and visible, so she creates a checklist on her calendar. She loves checking things off each week and feeling like she accomplished something.

I love Sarah for her checklists and calendars, and I encourage you to follow her lead. Treat your healthy habits like you would treat a business meeting or a doctor's appointment. Write it down and give it the respect it deserves.

STEP 2: MOTIVATION

We know motivation isn't permanent. That's why the 12 Reasons exercise from Chapter 1 is so important. To make a sustained effort, you need to know your *real why* inside and out. In fact, there's even a space on your SMARTER Goals worksheet for you to write it down and remind yourself.

Why is this so important? Because on the inevitable day that you don't feel like exercising for thirty minutes—even though you planned for it—you'll have that *real why* ready to give you that extra kick in the pants to get going. Once you connect your *real why* with a specific goal, you're going to be a lot more likely to stick to it.

George Sets Out on Mission: Possible

George's knee is aching. "Must be a storm coming," he says to no one in particular. Maybe today isn't such a great day to go for that walk he was planning.

Then George remembers his *real why*. "If I exercise and lose weight, my knee is going to hurt less." The walk is out, but he decides to go swimming at the local health center instead. It doesn't cost him much, and swimming is the perfect kind of exercise for someone with a bum knee. He didn't give up on the overall goal (being healthier); he simply adjusted his plan when he had a barrier.

The thing George didn't expect is that, after he's done, he really *does* feel a lot better. He's one day closer to physical freedom—and now he's excited to keep going tomorrow!

STEP 3: ACTION PLAN

You already got a taste of how the action plan works when we talked about specific goals. It's a lot better to say, "I'm going to exercise for thirty minutes, three times a week" than to say "Gosh, it sure would be nice to exercise."

The more specific, the better. Get out your calendar and block out your time. For instance, maybe every Sunday afternoon you get groceries and chop vegetables. If you can visualize the activity and plan ahead for it, then you're far more likely to follow through.

Bill Is the Man with the Plan

While he's still on the fence about how much effort he's going to put into a healthier lifestyle, Bill has been meaning to get more exercise anyway, so now is a good time to throw himself into it.

This is where Bill's business acumen kicks in. Bill wants to know the who, what, when, and where of his workout routine. First, he grabs his calendaring app on his phone and starts blocking out the times—Monday, Wednesday, and Friday. Then, he starts planning the specifics. Bill likes a little variety in his life, so he builds that into his exercise schedule. On Mondays, he'll use that treadmill he bought five years ago. Wednesday, he'll go walking with his sons. Friday, his whole family will have fun with some workout videos he found on YouTube.

If Bill is anything, he's a dedicated servant to his calendar. Now that he has a concrete action plan, Bill realizes that a healthier lifestyle is a lot easier to pursue than he thought.

CAN YOU GET TOO SPECIFIC?

At this point, you may be wondering if there's a point where being too specific might actually hurt a goal? For instance, if your goal is to exercise three times a week and your action plan is to do that at the YMCA on Monday, Wednesday, and Friday at 5:30, what happens when your car breaks down or your membership expires?

If that happens, no sweat. This is why your SMARTER Goals worksheet moves from big-picture goal to specific-action plan. If you can't perform your specific activity, just back up a step. You may not be able to go to the Y, but you *can* still get your half hour of exercise in for the day some other way. You can still be a healthier person that day.

As long as you plan ahead and remember what your bigger-picture goals are, it's easy to pivot to plan B when necessary.

STEP 4: ROADBLOCKS

No matter how well you build out your action plan, something will disrupt your routine at some point. A ruptured disc in my back kept me from jogging for months. The hospital food I ate while recovering from appendicitis got me way off my normal eating plan for a time. Muffins are going to happen (remember those?).

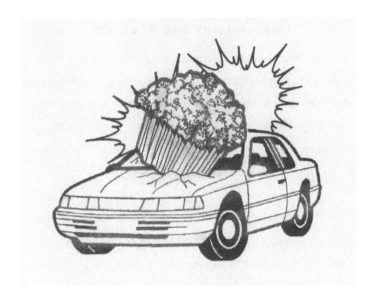

The question is, what are you going to do about them? At this part of the SMARTER Goals worksheet, your job is to list all the roadblocks that could get in the way of you and your goal. Maybe work will leave you too tired. Maybe your kids will get sick. Maybe you'll sprain your ankle. Maybe you'll be abducted by aliens.

On the left side of your paper, jot down as many possible roadblocks you can think of—no matter how big or how small. To the right of each roadblock, write down what you're going to do if it happens. How are you still going to get to your goal? If, for instance, those aliens totally derail your exercise routine, let them know they can study human physiology better if they let you use their treadmill.

If you're having trouble with this step, get on Facebook and find the Habit That Tribe. I or someone else on there is sure to have a suggestion for how you might get around this.

Sarah Turns Roadblocks to Road Pebbles

Sarah has a bunch of stuff to do. Right now, she's holding a screaming baby in one arm, while trying to help her other daughter glue together a diorama of outer space with the other hand. Getting those thirty minutes of exercise is the last thing on her mind.

But Sarah doesn't want to let these roadblocks stop her. "My goal was to exercise three times a week," she says. "I had planned it for today, but that's not happening. If I make time for it tomorrow, though, I'm still on pace to reach my goals for the week, month, and year."

Then another idea hits her. The screaming baby will tire out soon enough and fall asleep. Then she'll have time with her other daughter to focus on the outer space project. What if she and her daughter enhance their study time by inventing an outer space dance? Can't that be exercise, too?

Some roadblocks are easy to sidestep, while others will take a little creativity to get around. Sarah has given herself permission to adjust. She is firm on her exercise goal but flexible in how she's going to get there.

STEP 5: TIMETABLE

We all need deadlines. It's just the truth. I never would have finished this book if I didn't have plenty of deadlines along the way.

You want your deadlines to be both ambitious and realistic. Two sit-ups a year, for instance, is plenty realistic, but not very ambitious. On the other hand, two thousand sit-ups a day is plenty ambitious, but not very realistic. You need to find that middle ground.

That middle ground is going to be different for everyone. At marketing guru Joe Polish's Genius Network Annual Event, I saw Randi Zuckerberg tell an audience that her goal was to do 40,000 burpees in a year, which I thought was insane.[7] But, as she told us, she was able to keep that goal within reach by breaking it into smaller goals and then choosing her moments. Upon hearing this, Joe, another burpee aficionado, challenged Zuckerberg to a burpee-off.

---

7   Here, I have to admit that I guessed the number a little bit. Maybe it was 40,000 burpees, maybe it was 45,000, or maybe it was some other number entirely. I wasn't able to track down any video from the GN meeting, and I don't exactly have Randi on speed dial (though it sure would be pretty sweet if I did). Either way, her goal was to do a lot of burpees, and I was impressed by her ambition! To learn more about her efforts, search "Randi Zuckerberg burpees" on YouTube, and you'll see what I'm talking about. She's a great example of someone setting goals and sticking to them in multiple areas of her life.

Like the amazing woman that she is, she took off her heels, got the audience to participate as well, and then soundly beat everyone right there on stage—and in a dress, no less!

Randi Zuckerberg is now my hero.

Whatever deadline you set, be it a week, month, or year, ask yourself what you can do today to reach that goal. For instance, one of my current goals is to exercise three times a week for an entire year. That equals 156 workouts. So, I put a sheet on my wall with 156 blank boxes. Every time I exercise, I check one off.

You may find it's easier to stick with the weekly or monthly goals. Nothing wrong with that. Just be sure to set up those check boxes or other reminders each week/month to make sure you keep at it.

Also, make sure your goals are action-based, not result-based. It might sound like a good idea to say, "I'm gonna lose twenty pounds by this date," but you don't know how your body is going to respond to your new routine. Besides, depending on what you're doing to exercise, keep in mind that you'll likely be *gaining* muscle mass, meaning that although your body is getting healthier, you're not losing as much weight in some instances. Focus on the action and remember that your big-picture goal is to be a healthy person, and the results will follow.

Mary Maps Out a Plan

Mary has lived a life of somedays. Finally, she has decided that someday is *today*. Mary has thought about what she wants, she's considered her options, and now she's ready to start making decisions.

Feeling empowered, Mary sits down to map out her plan. She figures out what she's going to do, when she's going to do it, and how often she'll do it. Every now and then, she pauses, looks at herself in the mirror, and says, "I can absolutely do this. I can still have time to read books, knit, and hang out with my friends. I can check off those boxes, and then I can check off my healthy living boxes and feel good about myself."

Mary knows she's not running a 5K tomorrow, but she might someday. She'll start by walking a mile five times a week. Once she's done that for a month, she'll graduate to something harder and set a new timeline.

STEP 6: EVOLVE AND EVALUATE

"At the age of sixty-five, my grandma started walking five miles a day. She's ninety-two now. We have no idea where she is."

When I hurt my back, I couldn't do much physically. I definitely couldn't lift weights or run. I had to evolve my expectations and my practice. All I could do for a while was take walks—slow, agonizing walks, during which I felt that a senior citizen with a walker could outpace me—so that's exactly what I did. Sure, I wanted to do more. I felt super impatient all throughout my recovery and wanted desperately to push myself harder. However, I knew that if I did, I would hurt myself worse and would be out even longer. (How do I know this? Because I did it and set myself back—ugh!) Despite my frustration at the slowness of my progress, I was still able to check boxes and keep working toward my goals.

You will have to evolve and evaluate your habits, too. I knew someone who decided she was going to exercise every day for a year. It was too ambitious, and she found pretty quickly that she had to step back and reconsider. I've known other people whose goals were too easy, so they had to step them up. Either way, it's better to evolve the goal than to set something completely unrealistic, fail at it, and then quit because you see yourself as a failure. The thing is, you *can't* be a failure, no matter what you do. As Zig Ziglar often reminds us, "Failure is an event, not a person."

Whatever the case, remember that the only thing set in stone on your SMARTER Goals worksheet is the line at the very top: "I want to get healthier." That one is carved in granite. The rest are written in pencil.

Bill Shouldn't Weight Around

When he first gets to the gym, Bill heads straight to the free weights. Considering his heart attack, he should also be trying something more cardio-focused. But weights are what Bill knows, so weights are what Bill will do.

Bill hurts himself pretty quickly. He hasn't been in the weight room in a long, long time. He has no business even looking at the fifty-pound weights. The second he pulls a back muscle lifting one up, his body makes sure he's aware of this fact.

If he wants, Bill can make that fifty-pound weight his end goal. For now, Bill has to start where he has to start. At the moment, all he's got in him are a handful of push-ups and some curls. *That's fine for now*, he decides, *but not forever*. Bill is used to winning. He's going to learn from this experience, refocus on what he should be doing for his heart health, and commit to doing better.

Eventually, Bill will come to see these early struggles as part of his ultimate triumph. He's already been a rags-to-riches story with the business he's built. Now he's going to create a similar path for his health.

STEP 7: RECORD AND REWARD

You are what you measure. If you record it, you're more

likely to do it. If you reinforce that behavior with a reward, you're more likely to *keep* doing it. Let's looks at these one at a time.

First, Record

Right now, I want you to stop reading, grab a piece of paper, and create a visual checklist that will help keep you on target.

If you're like me and trying to exercise three days a week, put twelve boxes on your fridge each month. Or, if your goal is to complete exercises three times a week for a whole year, put 156 boxes on there. When I make a goal like that, there are some weeks I do less than three and some weeks I do more than three. It all depends on a variety of factors. Whatever the case, it is the overall goal that is important, not whether you followed it perfectly each day.

Maybe you're not the pen-and-paper type. Maybe you're the smartphone type. You know the old saying, "There's an app for that?" Well, that's doubly true when it comes to healthy living. I've seen firsthand how much food-tracking and goal-tracking apps have helped shape people's healthy habits.

Another reason record and reward works is that it holds

you accountable. If you eat a bag of Skittles, you have to record it, just like you would anything else. But instead of shaming yourself, use it as motivation.[8] The next time you pick up that bag of Skittles, ask yourself if you really feel like recording that in your food journal for the day.

Maybe apps aren't your thing. Here's something even simpler. Take a picture of whatever you're about to eat. Then ask yourself how badly you want it. If you *do* want it, how much are you going to eat? Are you going to eat the whole cake, or just the slice?

Then, Reward

Now the fun part—setting up rewards for yourself along the way.

With rewards, be mindful of the reward you choose. Ask yourself in advance, "What would make me feel good, and what do I feel like I want as a result of this?"

For me, I rewarded my jogging goal with a new pair of running shoes. I'd never been much of a runner, but now that I'd reached a milestone, I'd begun to see myself as

---

8 Here is a friendly public service announcement: shame does *not* burn calories. It simply burns your soul. If you struggle with shame, I suggest checking out the work of shame researcher Brene Brown, either through her books or her super-inspiring TED Talk. Either way, the bottom line is that shame isn't doing you any favors—and letting go of it will be a huge weight off your shoulders.

one. The shoes reinforced this new positive label and gave me an extra boost to keep building this good habit. Plus, I'm sure the bright color makes me run faster. My kids insist this is true with their light-up shoes!

Generally, I'd recommend against using food as a reward. If you do, though, tie it in with a different reward. For instance, maybe you're going to a party later in the month where you know the host makes killer nachos. Let the party—and all the nachos you can eat—be your reward for the month. Next month, reward yourself with something different.

WHAT REWARDS DO YOU USE?

The rewards you use should change and evolve. They don't need to be elaborate, either. Your reward could be as simple as designated alone time to reflect, replenish, or read a book. Whatever reward resonates with you, that's what you should do.[9]

Sarah Plans for a Night In

Sarah has set up a calendar on her fridge with twelve exercise boxes for the month. Once they're all checked, she's going to do something loving and replenishing for herself.

---

9   It's always fun to learn what other people do to reward themselves. Join the HabitThat Tribe on Facebook to share your unique rewards and see what other people are doing.

Maybe she'll get a babysitter and enjoy a fun evening out with people she loves, or maybe she'll treat herself to a nice, long bath, a glass of wine, and a good book. She's already got her milestone mapped out for next month, too.

Seeing what she's going to do—and what she's going to give herself—helps Sarah's goals feel real. She's excited about reaching every step along the way, and the pursuit of a reward has even made the process fun.

George High-Steps to Disneyland

George wants to record how many steps he's taking every day. He also wants to hit his goal of making it to the pool at least once a week. He *needs* to do this because otherwise he won't have the stamina to enjoy his reward: a vacation to Disneyland with his grandkids.

If he's going to Disneyland, George wants to do it right. He wants to be able to walk around, wear some Mickey Mouse ears, enjoy the rides, and spoil his grandkids. His granddaughter is getting a magic fairy wand for sure, and his grandson won't stop talking about how many churros he's going to eat.

But after that vacation, what's next? George's reward has a specific date. He's going to need another reward to keep going, perhaps future vacations with his grandkids—maybe something even more ambitious, like a two-week trip to Europe!

THE MAGIC OF MOTIVATIONAL POSTERS

There's a quote I like to share when I'm giving my Behavior Change workshops to future doctors. "The less definite and immediate the consequences, the less likely you are to change."

First, I show it as black words on a white slide, and everybody stares at me. Then, I click forward to the next slide. It has the exact same inspirational message, but now it's in front of a beautiful sunset and made up like a meme.

"Is this inspiring to you now?" I ask. Everybody laughs—and then they write the quote down. I get the same reaction every time.

Nevertheless, this quote perfectly embodies why I like the SMARTER Goals exercise and why I think it works. The more real you make your goals, the more likely you will be to act on them.

THE SMARTER GOALS WORKSHEET

Now that you've learned every step of the SMARTER

process, it's almost time to start filling out your own work-sheets. A few more things, and then I'll let you get to it.

YOUR BIGGEST GOAL STAYS THE SAME

It doesn't matter who you are. Your biggest goal at the top of your worksheet is being a healthy person. I've already filled this part of the worksheet out for you. The work-sheet will guide you through the rest.

YOU'RE GOING TO HAVE MORE THAN ONE GOAL

You get one specific goal per sheet. For instance, your first goal might look like this:

Be healthy.

Lose weight.

Exercise thirty minutes, three days a week.

The next goal might start the same, but the specific action will be different:

Be healthy.

Get more sleep.

No electronics or screens one hour before bedtime.

Set an alarm for screen-free time.

Each goal needs to be its own SMARTER process, because each will present different needs, roadblocks, or timelines.

DON'T OVERWHELM YOURSELF

Eventually you're going to end up with a lot of goals, but I don't want you to be overwhelmed. Take those goals one at a time. If you're not sure where to start, I've provided a few options on my website (www.drhopehealth.com).

Remember, you start where you start. If five minutes is all you have each day, then don't set up ten goals. Start with something you know you can manage, grow it into a habit, and then decide your next step from there. And if five minutes really is all you have, that's great! I can't emphasize enough that five minutes is better than no minutes. If you can do something that forwards your goal for even five minutes a day, the small changes *will* add up to big rewards.

I started off overwhelmed, too. Back then, I was a Cheetotarian. I ate nothing but junk food and didn't exercise much. I would stay up late, burn the candle at both ends, and do nothing to manage my mounting stress. The only veg in those days was all the time I spent vegging out in front of the TV. I also didn't feel very good most of the time. Overhauling my entire lifestyle wasn't going to happen overnight.

I didn't even know what goal to start with, so I just decided, "I wanna get healthy." It took me a while to figure out what that meant to me and how to approach it, but I knew that if I was going to become a physician and help others get healthier, I had to start somewhere. Plus, I wanted to look and feel better.

I started with drinking the recommended amount of water every day. That became my keystone habit. Once I was good at it, I moved on to adding more veggies to my diet (but not those evil green beans!). Then, I added exercise. The habits are now so ingrained, I don't have to think about it. It may take a while, but each step builds on the last, and you'll feel better as you go. Eventually, it will become ingrained into your lifestyle and be easier than you can imagine!

YOU DON'T HAVE TO OVERHAUL YOUR LIFE

When my wonderful yet mildly stubborn father-in-law decided to get healthy, life had just thrown him a big muffin. His wife, my mother-in-law, had been diagnosed with pancreatic cancer, and they had both come to live with us so they could be close to the hospital for her treatments and so we could help them on their journey.

My father-in-law wanted to be healthy enough to take care of his wife. He wasn't in a position to do anything more, even if he'd wanted to. To get there, he identified two goals within his reach: walk daily and eat a breakfast with protein. That was it—no dramatic changes, just two health-forward goals he knew he could fulfill.

Slowly but surely, my father-in-law lost sixty-five pounds, even as he sat for countless hours with his sick wife through every hospital stay, doctor visit, and chemotherapy treatment. His improved diet gave him the energy to support her, and the daily walks gave him the opportunity to clear his head.

When my mother-in-law passed, he had to find a new *real why*, but he kept going. He *had* to keep going. The pain of losing a spouse is immense, and the surviving partner needs to regroup. She told him many times that she wanted him to enjoy his life, and she taught all of us so many valuable lessons on appreciating the time we have. Before she got sick, they both loved to travel. So, these days, he is processing her loss in a healthy and proactive way. Instead of isolating himself and sitting at home, he is making specific efforts to get out of the house to see friends, family, and the world. His prior *why* was being healthy enough to take care of her. His new *why* is to be healthy enough to take care of himself and enjoy his precious time. The reason and the goals have changed, but he's been repeatedly able to evolve and evaluate. I am incredibly proud of him.

START SETTING YOUR SMARTER GOALS!

Okay, stop right there. Before reading any further, flip to Appendix C and start filling out some SMARTER Goals. Start with two or three, see how you feel, and then revise and add from there! Remember, motivation isn't permanent—so if you are feeling it right now, take advantage of it! Motivation is what gets you started, but habits are what keep you going. And you care about healthy habits because you've made it this far already! What will your keystone habit be?

For examples of others' SMARTER Goals, check out www.drhopehealth.com.

YOUR STORY STARTS NOW

You've heard from our patients. You've heard from me. You've heard from my father-in-law. You've even written your own SMARTER Goals using the worksheet in Appendix C to help get you going. Now it's time to start telling your own story.

As you dive into the SMARTER Goals worksheet and then into Part II of the book, here's a quick reminder. You already have a ton of good habits in your life, even if they're just simple things like brushing your teeth and getting dressed every day. You're already using these habits to your advantage. Now it's time to build a few more.

Each keystone habit will get you to a healthier life. Even if you only have five minutes a day, that time will start accumulating into a big impact on your life.

Even if you exercise five minutes a day, that's 1,825 minutes a year more than you were doing! Living healthier doesn't have to only mean going to the gym for an hour, five days a week. All it means is changing one habit at a time for the better.

Maybe you're the all-in type or maybe you're the slow-and-steady type. Whatever the case, set your goals to match who you are and what you're realistically capable of.

Think of yourself as a snowball on top of the hill. As you start to roll down, you get bigger and bigger, building more momentum as you go. If you focus on each step of the journey and savor your quick wins, a year from now, you'll look back and be astonished at everything you've accomplished.

CONGRATULATIONS!

If change were easy, we would all be fit, none of us would be smokers, and we would all be managing our stress.

The Habit That lifestyle isn't easy—and neither is getting through the first half of a book! Seriously, I'm not making this up. A lot of people don't read the books they buy at all, let alone get past the first chapter. And yet here you are, all done with the first half and ready to keep going!

You've made it through the hard part. That's what healthy people do. Why not take a moment to reward yourself before moving on to Part II?

PART II

THE FOUR PILLARS OF HEALTH

CHAPTER 4

EAT

Remember my grandma's "Fat Ladies' Club?" She and her friends have been at it for twenty years. They don't eat the day of the weigh-in, and then they all eat a huge meal together afterward. Their hearts are in the right place, but their approach needs a little refining.

For whatever reason, they love having me as a guest speaker. I think they just like my energy and my goofiness. Plus, they all know I'm a doctor, and they love hearing my wild tales from the ER.

Usually, whatever story I tell, I try to tie it in with one of the four pillars of health—stress, sleep, exercise, and especially food. I never lecture or scold them, though. Instead, I give them the opportunity to share both with me and each other. "Here is a struggle a lot of people have," I'll say. "What do all of you think, and how have you overcome this struggle in particular?"

Many people come up with stuff that's amazing, many times things I never would have thought of—in fact, they helped me refine a lot of the approaches in this book to match people in the real world—and I really enjoy helping them help themselves.

However, like many of us, they still struggle with healthy eating habits. Whenever the conversation comes up, I make it my number-one job to give them permission to eat and nourish their bodies—and to feel good about themselves in the process.

WHY HEALTHY EATING IS SO IMPORTANT

"If you are what you eat, then are cannibals the only real humans?"

In case there was any doubt in your mind, or you're an aspiring breatharian (yes, that's a real pseudo-thing), you absolutely need food to survive. We're exposed to food almost as much as the air. It's all around us, and it's necessary for basic life functions.

Our bodies depend on us to feed them, but they also depend on us to keep our digestive systems in balance.

Here's how it works. The primary part of food absorption takes place in your small intestines, and the intestinal lining—the only thing between your food and the inside of your body—is a single cell-layer thick. That's thinner than a piece of tissue paper!

Now, imagine taking a burger, or something equally greasy, and rubbing it on your skin. It's all over your face, your arms, and all up and down your body. Sounds lovely, right? This is essentially what you're doing to the inside of your body whenever you eat, rubbing it up and down everywhere until it becomes a part of you.

Yes, the old cliché is true: you *are* what you eat.

Your body will do its best to extract anything it can out of the food you give it, even if it's empty calories. It may not like it, but it's in no position to be picky; your body needs calories and energy to survive. If you literally drink poison, your body will still take it in and try to find something to do with it. Don't hate on your intestines; they're just doing their job!

Whatever you take in, it heads down to your gut, where between four and seven hundred different species of (mostly) helpful bacteria live. Those bacteria digest our food as well as they can, and then get rid of the rest through our stool. All those bacteria are constantly shedding and regrowing, and the success of this process is directly linked to the quality of food we provide them.

I like to say it's like fishing. You put different things on your line to get a certain type of fish. If you put a shrimp on there, you're going to get one type of fish. If you put a worm on the line, you'll get another kind of fish.

Whichever types of foods you're feeding your bacteria, those types of bacteria are going to grow more. Some bacteria actually make us fatter because they preferentially break down and help you absorb more of the unhealthy food. Other bacteria are all about breaking down healthy food and extracting the maximum amount of nutrients, leaving very minimal waste behind. Which would you rather have more of? Choose to feed the one you want!

What all this comes down to is this: if you eat french fries every now and then, it won't make a huge difference in your gut flora. However, if you continue to eat french fries regularly, you'll start feeding the wrong bacteria— the neighborhood bullies instead of the good kids—and then the bullies are going to start to grow.

As I tell my grandma's weight loss club, I don't say any of this to guilt or shame anyone. I love eating, and I want you to, too!

That said, to build healthy habits, it's important to check in with yourself with whatever you're about to eat. Ask yourself:

- Do you *really* want to rub that food up and down inside your body?
- Do you *really* want it to become part of you?

Sometimes, healthy habits really are as simple as these little time-outs. After all, the time-outs worked for Zack Morris, so why can't they work for you?

SHAME ON SHAME!

During one of my grandma's weight loss group meetings, another member was encouraging the idea of food shaming. The shame food of that week, she said, was brownies. Anyone who had eaten a brownie in the last week had to stand up and be shamed.

This kind of stuff horrifies me.

Eating is fun. Eating socially is even more fun—and brownies are delicious! I happily overate at my family's most recent Thanksgiving, and I'll happily overeat at other points in my life, too. I can do this without guilt precisely because it is an *occasional* indulgence rather than a regular habit. It is easily balanced out by the good eating habits I maintain most other days.

We need to take the shame and guilt away from food! It leads to bad choices. Shame and guilt make old ladies starve themselves before weigh-ins. Shame and guilt drive us to hide in the bathroom with candy bars. Shame and guilt drive us to drink odd vinegar-and-baking-soda mixes so we lose our appetites and don't eat anything.

IF YOU SAY IT, YOU BELIEVE IT

Shame and guilt also lead to misinformation, and misinformation can be very difficult to combat. You've probably learned to put peroxide and rubbing alcohol in a wound, but the truth is that those substances actually impair your healing and make scars worse. Turns out, people are suffering the sting for no benefit!

Peroxide and rubbing alcohol may be a harmful myth, but it's a harmful myth most of us learned from someone we trusted. So when we hear stuff like that, we tend to believe it—and then to share it. Once we share it, we believe it even more. Soon, we're saying things like, "Yeah, I hear it all the time, so it's gotta be true."

That's how the fad diets start. Someone hears that avocados and nuts are fatty and cuts them out completely—yet still eats chips and cake. Someone else hears that cabbage soup is chock-full of nutrients and only eats that from now on. Someone else hears that rice cakes are a health food and builds a diet around that. (Spoiler alert, rice cakes are *not* a health food. We just think they are thanks to clever marketing and bullshit.)

Each of these fads is well-intentioned, but they miss the point. Instead of restricting your diet, I want to help you understand all the good things you can do and focus on that.

YOU'VE GOT THAT HANGRY FEELING

Because they've skipped meals before weigh-in, my grandma's club is always starving after a meeting. So, they all head out to a restaurant. First, one lady orders a burger, and then another. "Oh, this is a weight-loss club," one of them says, "and look at what we're doing!" They all laugh, and soon the whole table has ordered burgers.

When we feel bad about eating, we skip meals. And when we skip meals, our bodies start demanding high-energy foods ASAP.

I've gone through the different stages of hunger plenty of times at work. With those first hunger pangs, I start thinking about how good a salad sounds right now. Then, my body chemistry changes—specifically, I start to crave fat. By the end of the shift, if I still haven't been able to eat anything, I want the greasiest burger I can find. I want fries. I want cake. I want to eat the patient's arm next to me because I'm so hungry.

That's what we do to our bodies when we skip meals for too long. We go from "Yes, we're ready for nutrition" to "We need to survive. Eat a whole tube of cookie dough" really quickly.

Next, we begin to rationalize it. Our psychology has changed. "Well, if I'm craving it, my body must need it," we say. Healthy food literally doesn't taste as good at this point. Only the fattiest of fats will do.

Nothing good comes out of starving yourself. That "hangry" feeling is real. If you go too long without eating, first you will start to get grumpy, and then maybe even a little shaky. It's just your body's way of saying, "I need this, and you're ignoring this need."

NERD ALERT: THE SCIENCE OF BEING HANGRY

In a very simplified view of body chemistry, ghrelin is your hunger hormone—growlin' ghrelin, I call it. The hormone leptin does the opposite; it tells you when you're full. When your stomach is empty, your blood sugar is down, and your body is ready for another meal. So, it starts producing ghrelin. That stimulates your appetite.

Later on, when you're stuffed after Thanksgiving, your ghrelin level goes down and leptin does its thing. Even if someone puts your favorite food in front of you, you won't want it. It won't even smell as good. You don't need it.

The cycle repeats. As you get hungrier again, your ghrelin starts going up and suddenly that same food you were waving away earlier smells fantastic. That's your body's way of telling you it's time to eat—much in the same way your bladder tells you it's time to pee.

But just like we ignore signals that we need to pee because we are oh so busy, we ignore signals that we're hungry. The longer you go, the more your body goes into famine mode. "Oh crap, we're not going to eat," it says. "Next meal, we'd better store every single calorie because who knows how often food is coming?"

Now, most of us have more than enough stored fat, sugar, and energy. We've got supplies if we need to go a few hours without eating. That's not good enough for your body. It wants a regular supply of energy to feel secure. It's a big worrywart that way.

When you're this super hungry, you also want to eat as fast

as possible. This leads to overeating. If you eat too fast, you're full before your body realizes you're full. It takes a bit for your stomach to realize it's reached capacity and that it needs to shut off the ghrelin and pump up the leptin. Sometimes, we continue to eat even when our bodies have said enough, and we end up moaning in misery on the couch after Thanksgiving dinner.

In other words, pay attention to what your body is telling you—and as early as possible. If you catch those hunger pangs early, you won't feel like snapping at everyone and eating everything in sight. And if you eat slowly, you'll be more attuned to your body telling you when to stop.

THIS IS HOW YOU HABIT THAT

Most people I know want to eat healthy. They'd love to be making 90 percent healthy food choices and 10 percent indulgent ones. That's a great goal, but it's also not the reality for many of us, who are usually about 50/50 (or sometimes worse) when it comes to our food choices. By focusing on the following healthy eating habits, we can start to shift the balance more toward that 90/10 ideal.

PLAN MEALS IN ADVANCE

When you plan what you're going to eat in advance, you know what you'll have available. The less you leave to chance, the better. It's hard to go into a gas station and purchase a healthy meal. But if you pack some healthy snacks, perhaps some chopped veggies or nuts, then it's much easier to make healthy choices throughout the day.

You can also plan your indulgences in advance. If you know Friday is going to be pizza night, you'll be more likely to make healthy choices Monday through Thursday. And then when Friday comes around, you can enjoy yourself because you've been eating healthy all week. If I plan to go out with my girlfriends, we'll have wine and maybe a delicious dessert. I eat healthy for the rest of the week and don't binge even when I enjoy my indulgences. This makes the unhealthy 10 percent fun and guilt-free, while the healthy 90 percent keeps me on track for my goals.

CREATE ROUTINES

Now that you've planned ahead, it's time to execute. And that means routines. Friday is pizza night (with a side salad to go with it). Every second Wednesday is drinks with coworkers. Sunday is veggie-chopping day.

Following a routine reduces your cognitive load. That is, once you've created a routine, it becomes automatic. You don't have to think about it. This frees your mind up for important stuff like work, family games, and the random song lyrics that pop into your brain unexpectedly. This is important, because motivation isn't permanent. It's hard to make good decisions when you get home if you've already been making tons of other decisions all day.

Routines help you make good decisions when you're in the right mindset. That way, when you're in the wrong mindset later, you get to rely on the good, strong choices you made earlier, rather than the exhausted, hangry choices you feel like making in the moment.

BRING SNACKS

My body has to survive somehow during those ten- or twenty-four-hour ER shifts. If a patient is crashing, I can't just say, "Hold on. Everybody stop. I need a salad."

That's why I stash a protein bar, some nuts, or some cut-up vegetables somewhere close by. It gives me immediate convenience food that I can eat between patients or while filling out paperwork. I also usually bring a green smoothie (my favorite mix is kale, spinach, turmeric, blueberries, raspberries, and pineapple) so I can drink my fruits and veggies on the go. After all, it's hard to sit for a proper four-course meal when you have to treat a waiting room full of people!

People have definitely teased me about my healthy food stashes. I'm like a squirrel. But invariably, whenever they get hungry, they ask, "Uh, can I have some of your snacks?"

My kids do the same thing. As soon as we get in the car, they ask, "What are we having?"

Through my own habits, I have unwittingly created a habit for them. I've associated my car with snacks. Instead of fighting it, I roll with it. Whoever asks for snacks gets chopped vegetables, peppers, pea pods, and stuff like that. If we're going to create a snacking habit in the car, it will be a healthy snacking habit. (My poor kids! But don't report me just yet: they *do* get actual treats sometimes, too.)

ALLOW YOURSELF TREATS

Treats are great. But let them be exactly what they're supposed to be—treats.

I don't eat a brownie every day, but when I do, I take my time with it. Many a friend and colleague has heard me say, "Excuse me, but I'm going to need a moment alone with this brownie."

The way I see it, eat it fast if you don't like it, but eat it slow if you do. It will make your treat feel extra treat-y. That way, you really do get to have your cake and eat it, too!

WATCH OUT FOR THE SUGAR CRASH

Snickers has made a mint off their "hangry moment" commercials. I'm sure you've seen at least one or two. They'll start with a well-known celebrity being moody. Then someone hands them a Snickers, and they turn back into decent human beings again.

It's a great campaign because it's relatable. However, although Snickers has some fat and protein value with its peanuts, it's not something I would recommend as a regular snack.

Sugar creates a sugar need. When you eat sugar, you're riding a sugar high. Suddenly, you have tons of sugar and fat in your system. Responding to this sensory overload, your body releases a ton of insulin to balance out your system, and suddenly you experience a big energy crash.

When you crash, you start to feel sleepy and want to get your energy back. That's when most of us turn to more candy bars and energy drinks, but all this really does is keep the cycle going. It's a cycle of quick fixes that creates a long-term dependency.

This is why prepping and planning ahead is so helpful; it allows you to solve those hangry moments with nutrition. If healthy food isn't available to help perk you up, try something else instead, like taking a short walk.

RETHINK DAILY SERVINGS

We focus a lot on how many things we have to eat in a particular day. We need X servings of fruits and vegetables, X servings of protein, and X servings of healthy fats. Your body doesn't work exactly like that. Depending on what you're doing, it needs different things at different times.

Instead of looking at what you need every day, step it back. Just focus on getting enough vegetables, proteins, and healthy fats over the course of a week instead of a day. That way, if there's a day that it doesn't work out, perhaps because you're traveling, you've got the rest of the week to balance it out.

We live by the weekly system at our house. For instance, say we want to eat five servings of leafy greens, five servings of cruciferous vegetables, and five servings of other vegetables each week. We'll create a chart for the week, and each time we have one of those things, we check it off. This works just as well for drinking water or getting enough exercise. As we said last chapter, it's all about recording and rewarding.[10]

This helps with planning. If I know I have to eat X amount of veggies in a week, I'll plan my spots. I'll chop them

---

10   I've provided an example of what one of these goal-oriented worksheets might look like in Appendix D. For more examples—and even blank templates—head over to www.drhopehealth.com.

ahead of time so I can meet my goals on the go. Otherwise, it's going to be a lot harder to honor them.

Finally, with your weekly charts, don't worry about the foods you're limiting. Don't focus on what you don't want to do or what you can't have. Focus on what you *do* want to do by listing all the healthy things that you *are* going to do—the foods you'll feel empowered to eat and that help you reach your goals.

TOSS OUT THE FOOD PYRAMID

When people ask me how many servings they should have of different kinds of food, I keep it simple: vegetables are always good for you. I'm not saying you should become a vegetarian, just that these should be part of your diet every week.

Focus on cruciferous vegetables and leafy greens—the former for their active cancer-fighting properties and the latter because they have more ounce-for-ounce nutritional value than any other food available. Beans and lentils have a lot of positive health properties and can help decrease huge spikes in blood sugar. It's also okay to get regular servings of whole grains, such as millet, amaranth, quinoa, and barley if you don't have a sensitivity.

The government-sponsored food pyramid is now widely acknowledged to be inconsistent with healthy eating practices. Get rid of this old, outdated idea! It was based more on the influence of lobbying groups than on nutritional science. The fat-phobic simple-carb-heavy diet it created is well-known to increase health problems, including diabetes, heart attacks, and high cholesterol. While you should use unhealthy fats sparingly, such as those found in fried foods, feel free to stock up on healthy fats from nuts, avocados, olive oil, and fish regularly. Eating fat doesn't make you fat, but eating unhealthy, inflammatory, and highly processed foods and carbs can!

ENJOY HEALTHY FOODS, TOO

Yes, it is possible to enjoy yourself while eating healthy foods. No, seriously. Stop laughing.

Think about the satisfying crunch of a vegetable. If you're my kids, you chomp your veggies like a dinosaur. It's fun, satisfying, and you can enjoy the fresh taste, spices, and texture. Note: if you try this in a five-star restaurant, I suggest keeping the roaring and chomping to a minimum. Maybe pretend you're a fluffy woodland creature rather than a dinosaur.

Do the action, and the feeling will follow. Your taste buds *will* change with your habits.

As a kid, I hated every vegetable and wouldn't eat anything, but now I know food doesn't have to be covered in melted chocolate to be delicious. Today, I actually enjoy the taste of Brussels sprouts. I think they're delicious. A perfectly crisp apple with the right combination of sweet and crunchy is delicious. I genuinely look forward to my green smoothies every day. I still hate green beans, but hey, can't win 'em all, right?

People have an image in their head that they can eat nothing but rabbit food. They think everything has to be tasteless, dull, and otherwise awful in order to be healthy, but that's not true at all. There are so many fresh, wonderful, delicious things that you can enjoy—especially if you're willing to explore.

You should have seen me when I first began exploring healthier eating. I would go through phases where I put quinoa in everything. I would read an article about basil, and suddenly even my oatmeal had basil in it.

My family would roll their eyes on holidays when I'd try to sneak ground-up cauliflower into the cheesy potatoes. One time, they caught me putting black beans in brownies (which is actually really good).[11] It's gotten to the point

---

11   You want to know how to make it? Okay, I'll tell you how to make it. Start with a premade Ghirardelli chocolate brownie mix box, and then add one can of rinsed and blended smooth black beans (yup, from a can) and one can of water. Then, sprinkle in some unsweetened cocoa powder for extra chocolatey goodness, flax and chia, and some cinnamon. I'm not pretending it's a salad, but for a dessert, it's not the worst thing I could have! I think they taste great, and most of my victims—um, I mean friends and family—agree. *Warning:* if you don't eat a lot of beans at baseline, go easy on the brownies the first time, lest you end up learning the hard way. (I'm looking at you, Cindy!)

where, every time I bring a dish, they poke it suspiciously and say, "What's hiding in here? Is this real food, or something that *you* made?"

It's great that they indulge me, and it's also great that they're honest—each in their own way. If one of my experiments doesn't work, my dad will smile big and say, "This tastes really healthy, honey." Meanwhile, my mom will be at the other end, lovingly saying, "This tastes like ass! You need to *not* serve this to regular humans." You've got to love having both kinds of people in your life.

The family jokes reinforce my healthy eating goals because they allow me self-awareness. For a recent birthday, for instance, my mom made Texas sheet cake—one of my favorites—which is basically butter and flour holding a bunch of sugar and chocolate together. Whenever she serves it to me, she always jokes, "I didn't make any black beans. There's no cauliflower in here. It's just cake."

And what great cake it is.

BE MINDFUL OF FOOD SHAMERS

Not everyone will be as supportive as my family. You might have friends who aren't ready to change—perhaps because they're struggling with their own healthy habits— and they might get mean about it.

This is a real roadblock you will likely face, so it's helpful if you can identify who these people might be in advance. If you're the only one in your group making healthy choices, the group might single you out with nasty comments.

It's hard to be around that. Most of your friends will celebrate your Habit That lifestyle, but one or two won't. If it's hard to eat around them, remove the negative opportunity. Do activities with those people where food isn't the focus, like seeing a movie, going shopping, or taking a walk.

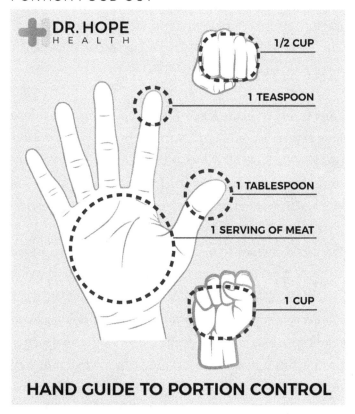

DR. HOPE
H E A L T H

1/2 CUP

1 TEASPOON

1 TABLESPOON

1 SERVING OF MEAT

1 CUP

HAND GUIDE TO PORTION CONTROL

Food portioning is a lot more important than you might realize—both for healthy and unhealthy foods. If you decide that you're going to have some chips, decide how many you're going to eat. That way, you won't eat the whole bag.

Maybe you've been to an expensive restaurant and heard someone complain, "For such an expensive restaurant, this is a tiny portion." The funny thing is, whatever's on your plate is probably an appropriate serving size. That's about how much a normal human is supposed to eat. The supersize culture has tricked us into unnecessarily large portions.

Your stomach is the size of your fist. Seriously, take a look at your fist right now. Not that impressive, is it? Now imagine stuffing a thirty-two-ounce steak into your fist—or perhaps a giant coffee shop muffin or a whole bag of chips. Those aren't single servings—more like four or five!

First, take a week to become conscious of serving size. Take the time to read packages. It will be a crazy reality check. Then, keep eating as many vegetables as you want. For everything else, start reading labels or doing a bit of reading to understand appropriate serving sizes, learn to portion the right amounts out, and commit to only eating that much. Put the rest away. There's no need to challenge your willpower with temptation.

Nerd Alert: Portion size prowess in the palm of your hand.

Portion sizes can be confusing, especially in today's supersized world! That coffeehouse muffin you are eating might be as many as 4 servings depending on the size. And who eats half a muffin anyway? As you get more savvy, you will remember to look at packages for serving size, you will be surprised at how few chips, candies, or treats constitute one serving, yet the bag seems suspiciously like something you want to finish in one sitting. As your habits improve, you will be eating less things from bags and boxes anyway. So how much should you eat? Do you need to carry around scales and fancy informercial gadgets?? Nope! All you need is in the palm of your hand...

> **3 ounces:** the recommend serving size for meat is the size of the palm of your hand
> **1 cup:** Approximately the size of your clenched fist
> **1 oz:** your thumb (think things you want to limit, such as cheese)
> **1 teaspoon:** the tip of your thumb
> **1-2 oz:** Snacks that fit in the palm of your hand (like almonds)

When it comes to serving sizes, the unhealthier foods should get the smallest size in your days. The healthier foods, especially vegetables, should get top billing. Here are some general guidelines:

> **Meat/Fish/Egg/Dairy:** 3 oz serving
> **Vegetables:** 5-7 1 cup servings daily, aim to have varied types such as greens, crucifers, and others
> **Fruits:** 2-3 1 cup servings daily, aim to include berries
> **Beans/Lentils:** 1-3 ¼ to ½ cup size servings per day

OTHER TRICKS:

· **Use a smaller plate:** it will make your portion size seem larger & trick your eyes.
· When eating out, if they give big portion sizes, **ask for a box at the beginning of the meal** and keep only one serving on your plate so you aren't tempted to overeat while you are socializing
· **Eat slowly,** give your stomach time to realize that it is getting full so it can send you the right signals before you are stuffed
· **Chew your food:** your stomach does not have teeth. Take the time to enjoy it, the tastes, the textures, and improve your digestion at the same time.

BE DONE WHEN YOU'RE DONE

When we were younger, my brother used to eat until he was stuffed and uncomfortable. He thought that was how he was supposed to feel when he was done eating. In reality, he was just training his body to ignore the feeling of being full.

I train my kids to be members of the Anti-Clean Your Plate Club. At every meal, I tell them, "If your body says it's done, be done" (unless they are trying to apply this to their vegetables, of course). They have literally stopped mid-pancake at breakfast when their tummies were full. This is different from what I was told growing up. "Finish your plate. There's starving kids in the world" (to which I usually replied I'd be happy to send them my food—especially my green beans). This mindset is ingrained in most of us, and it's not easy to break.

Remember, it takes time for your body to tell you that it's full. Your body needs a bit to make a hormone, pump it into your blood, and send it to your brain.

This is why slowing down is one of the most basic healthy goals you can make. Even healthy eaters don't eat slowly enough. Remember, your stomach has no teeth, so don't be afraid to chew your food more thoroughly.

Chewing slowly also gives your body the time to stimulate saliva production, which tells your body that you've started eating. When you slow down, you realize that you're full when you're *actually* full, instead of getting the message too late like my brother would. He's reformed his habits, and if a stubborn mule like him can (love you, Roger!), you can too!

PREPARE FOR CRAVINGS

Even something as simple as the smell of food can pit our cravings against us. I worked at a movie theater as a teenager, and management specifically instructed us to make fresh popcorn even if we had more than enough—just because people are drawn to the smell of popcorn in the air.

By midafternoon most days, I crave chocolate. Other people I know crave a cookie after dinner. If you're like that too, that's fine. Just plan for it in advance and control the portion.

Sometimes smelling something is enough. If you peel and eat a fresh orange, the smell of the citrus stimulates some of the "happy" receptors in your brain, reminding your body of sunshine and feeling healthy. When I'm at a restaurant, I love taking in the scent of a juicy burger and crisp fries. But instead of giving in to my hangry brain, I simply let myself enjoy the moment and then order something that won't leave me feeling bloated and sluggish later.

Another thing to do when you're experiencing a craving—or even if you're mid-binge—is to redirect it. For instance, chocolate doesn't taste good after eating an orange. Don't have an orange? Go brush your teeth. Nothing tastes good after that.

Here are some other simple tips: drink a big glass of water. Go for a walk or distract yourself for ten or fifteen minutes to see if a little perspective helps. Most likely, you'll find your craving won't be as bad once the triggering food isn't staring you in the face.

NERD ALERT: ARE YOUR GENES TO BLAME?

Some people like to blame their genes when it comes to diet and weight gain. But even stubborn genes can be trained. Yes, your genes do determine certain traits of your body, but they don't determine whether you're a healthy or unhealthy person. Easy example: identical twins have the same genes, right? Imagine you had an identical twin and one of you ate nothing but junk food, while the other one managed diet and stress. Who do you think is going to look better in five years?

Your genes produce proteins based on the messages they receive. If you send them the message that you are stressed, your genes will help your body produce survival hormones such as cortisol, and your body will store fat as a way to pad from stress. Thus, when you are highly stressed, it is harder to lose weight. If you manage stress and eat the same foods, your body isn't getting the "store for protection" messages, and you will look different. Now, imagine the benefits of managing your stress *and* eating healthier foods. That sends the message to your genes that things are well in your world, and you can let go of excess weight and feel great!

You have more power over your genes than you think you do. Whatever messages you tell your genes, they will listen— even if they're a little reluctant at first. So, what message do you want to tell them?

HOW DIET AFFECTS YOUR BODY

People think about food as something that makes them sad. They're sad when it makes them gain weight. They're sad when they have to eat healthy. They're sad either way. That makes me so sad to see all this sadness associated with the wonders of food!

Do the habit, and the good feeling will follow. Your diet directly affects your body's internal environment (remember the image of rubbing your food all over your insides?), and you are a reflection of that environment. Many of America's biggest health concerns—depression, fatigue, anxiety—are directly linked to an unhealthy diet. Fortunately, your body reflects a healthy diet, too. Let's take a look at how.

IT'S ALL ABOUT INFLAMMATION

If you get a sunburn and your skin turns a bit red, that's inflammation. If you sprain your ankle and it swells, that's inflammation. When your body is exposed to some form of damage, it sends out the cleanup crew, which leads to inflammation.

This doesn't just happen with injuries. When you eat inflammatory foods, you create damage along the lining of your gut. Meanwhile, your blood vessels get coated with fat plaques that can lead to heart attacks and strokes. Your inflammatory crew needs to take care of these, too, but if it's busy cleaning up all the time from unhealthy food choices, it has fewer resources to fight off other diseases and infections.

Here's the other thing: anti-inflammatory pills don't work. It's not just vitamin C that keeps you healthy, but also all of the other things in oranges or broccoli that help your body absorb vitamin C naturally. You can't pill your way into health. You actually have to eat healthy foods.

Stock Up on Anti-inflammatory Foods

Inflammation isn't that great. It leaves you feeling achy, tired, and grumpy. Plus, you're more likely to experience depression and anxiety or to develop irritable bowel syndrome, arthritis, and other joint issues.

People often want the quick fix. They think they can just eat junk and then take a probiotic, but it doesn't work that way. If your lawn is completely filled with weeds, throwing a few healthy grass seeds out there is not going to make much of a difference. You've got to get rid of the weeds.

Fortunately, there are plenty of anti-inflammatory foods to help out your natural cleaning crew. Aside from the oranges and broccoli I mentioned, I advise you to eat as many veggies as you want, along with nutrient-rich food like salmon, avocados, and nuts.

You'd be amazed how fast inflammation goes away just by changing your diet. Eating well really can do wonders for your body. It literally changes your body's chemistry, which in turn changes the way you feel.

TOP INFLAMMATORY FOODS

When people ask me about the inflammatory foods they should be avoiding, I share with them my Dirty Dozen:

1. Soda and energy drinks
2. Smoked foods and meats
3. Hydrogenated oils (soy, sunflower, safflower, "vegetable" oils)
4. Trans fats (found in margarine and many commercial baked goods)
5. Fried foods
6. White sugar

7. Synthetic Frankenfoods (chemical creations made for food longevity)
8. Refined processed bleached flour
9. Excess alcohol
10. Fast food
11. Processed/cured meat
12. Certain types of dairy

These foods can increase your risk for cancer, heart attacks, diabetes, stroke, and other badness. Scary, right? To reduce your risk, either avoid these foods or keep consumption to a minimum.

TOP ANTI-INFLAMMATORY FOODS

Now, I know what you're thinking, trusted Habit That Tribe member: "If I can't have all these yummy foods, then what *can* I have?" Great news! There are *tons* of foods that aren't so inflammatory or damaging as the Dirty Dozen. Here are thirteen of my favorites, ranging from mildly inflammatory or neutral to strongly anti-inflammatory:

1. Berries
2. Spices
3. Leafy greens
4. Cruciferous vegetables
5. Avocados

6. Green tea
7. Omega-3 fats (walnuts, wild-caught fatty fish)
8. Colorful fruits and vegetables
9. Chia seeds and flaxseeds
10. Flavorful roots such as garlic, onions, ginger, and turmeric
11. Cocoa powder (think dark chocolate with minimal sugar)
12. Beans and lentils
13. Nuts and seeds

That's right, you can enjoy plenty of delicious real food. Emphasis on real. If you're not sure, follow the "rot rule:" if the food can rot (fruits, vegetables) relatively quickly, it is not filled with preservatives and chemicals and is thus usually a good choice. If your food could survive the zombie apocalypse (I'm looking at you, Twinkies), it's best to avoid it.

DIAGNOSE YOURSELF: ARE YOU INFLAMMATORY?

When you eat unhealthily, all those foods tell your body messages that it's in an inflammatory environment, that food is not readily plentiful, and that it needs to store every type of calorie it takes in. No matter what you eat, actually, your food sends your body messages, and your body responds.

If you're only putting garbage in, you can only feel like garbage, because that's all that is available.

If you're unsure whether you're in an inflammatory state, ask yourself if you have any of the following symptoms:

- Fatigue
- Chronic aches
- Arthritis
- Irritable bowels
- Depression
- Bad skin
- Stubborn fat around your midsection

If you answered in the affirmative to any of those symptoms, the next thing to do is take a look at how many inflammatory foods are in your diet. Although you could have underlying medical conditions as well (in which case, see your doctor!), many of these symptoms should improve with good healthy lifestyle habits.

FIGHTING CANCEROUS CELLS

Some types of foods have known carcinogens in them, meaning they are known to cause cancer. Once in your body, carcinogens move deep into your cells and damage your DNA. It's like someone walking into your kitchen and hitting your china cabinet. You can try to glue the pieces back together, but that cup's never going to work quite right again.

When cells get damaged, their DNA gets damaged—and if this happens in a particular way, the cells can turn cancerous and replicate uncontrollably. Your body has a very good cleanup system for fighting cancer, but sometimes that system can be overwhelmed or overcome. When that happens, the rogue cells grow into a tumor, and that tumor could become deadly.

Highly inflammatory food can cause cancer. Highly processed or smoked meats carry the biggest risk—another reason to limit how often you eat these kinds of foods. Every time you eat them, you introduce chemicals that can produce cancer cells in your body.

Your body may have the capacity to stop those cancer cells and kill them, but it all depends on how anti-inflammatory your body is and how well your genes can fight cancer. I say do everything you can to give it a fighting chance.

NERD ALERT: FROM SALIVA TO POOP—THE AMAZING JOURNEY OF YOUR FOOD

Your digestive system is a thirty-foot-long marvel of biological engineering! It takes anything you put into the mouth, digests and absorbs as much as possible, and discards the waste in a rather efficient manner, if things are working well. In the average lifetime, around sixty tons of food will pass through these precious pipes.

How long is the process, you ask? The remnants of the salad that you eat for lunch today will be flushed down the toilet likely sometime tomorrow or the following morning after your coffee. As it passes through you (gets rubbed all over your insides, that is), this is the journey it takes:

Mouth. This is your best opportunity to break down your food. There are no teeth elsewhere in your digestive tract, so let your mouth do its job. The mouth grinds, chops, and minces your food while adding saliva (up to 1.5 liters produced daily!) to lubricate it for the journey onward. Your mouth is the only part that can taste the yummy but unhealthy foods that might make it onto your plate. The rest of your GI system is *not* as easily impressed as your taste buds.

Esophagus. This ten-inch-long transit pipe connects your mouth to your stomach. When you swallow, it takes food about five to eight seconds to pass. Heartburn happens when the sphincter (like a door that opens and shuts at the connection between the esophagus and stomach) doesn't close tightly and acid from the stomach burns the more delicate lining of the esophagus. Overeating and being overweight make this sensation worse! Long term, acid reflux can cause scarring and even cancer in the esophagus.

Stomach. Your empty stomach is the size of your fist, but it can stretch. In fact, you have probably felt the stretch a little *too much* after certain holidays. The stomach is a mixing bag, churning your chewed food and adding in digestive acids. Your food spends about two to six hours here before it moves on to the intestines for absorption.

Small intestine. Measuring in at a whopping twenty-two feet with a surface area the size of a tennis court, your intestines are responsible for the majority of nutrient absorption. They are filled with billions and billions of bacteria that help your body digest the food and break down the nutrients for absorption. The gallbladder (if you still have one) and pancreas contribute additional digestive enzymes. Food can spend about three to five hours here as your body extracts nutrients (hint: give it healthy food!). Don't anger your intestines or you will feel the wrath of bloating and gas!

Colon. The large intestine is the slowest part of the GI tract. Here, water is absorbed and food starts to look (and smell!) more like poop. Depending on your colon health, level of hydration, and quality of the food you eat, food can be chillin' in the six-foot distance of your colon for anywhere from four to seventy-two hours, although neither of those extremes is ideal. Keep your colon healthy. To reduce your risk of colon cancer—the third leading cause of cancer-related deaths in men and women in the United States—make sure your colon is rubbed by healthy foods, fiber, plenty of water, and as few inflammatory foods as possible.

Toilet. Cheers to indoor plumbing! Congratulations, your salad has made it to its final destination. Your body has extracted all the nutrients that it could absorb, and now the remaining parts are indigestible fibers (which are good for you...like flossing your colon!), dead bacteria (they served bravely and valiantly in your guts and then followed your food out), mucus, and water.

Now that we've finished the journey, let's look at our poop to see how we did. Too much water in the stool equals diarrhea. Not enough equals constipation. Also, many medications affect your intestinal transit time, and antibiotics affect your gut bacteria.

Color matters, too. Your poop should be a deep brown color. Black and red are concerning, since they likely indicate bleeding somewhere in your intestinal tract (time to see your doctor). Pale stools can be a sign of inadequate digestive enzymes (again, see your doctor). Yellow can be a sign of a parasitic infection or problems with digestive enzymes (you already know what I'm going to recommend, don't you?). Blue is a sign of eating too many Smurfs, which you should definitely avoid.

As for shape, poop should be a long "log" and sink in the toilet. Floating stool can be a sign of too much fat, as well as poor nutrient absorption, and is usually associated with excessive gas.

Different diets lead to different kinds of poop. Diets rich in fruits, vegetables, and fiber lead to cleaner poop (less stuck to your butt, little to wipe away), so if you have to wipe a bunch of times, consider creating some SMARTER goals around vegetable intake!

Finally, if you aren't pooping nearly every day or if you have strangely colored or floating poops, you should (yup!) go see your doctor.

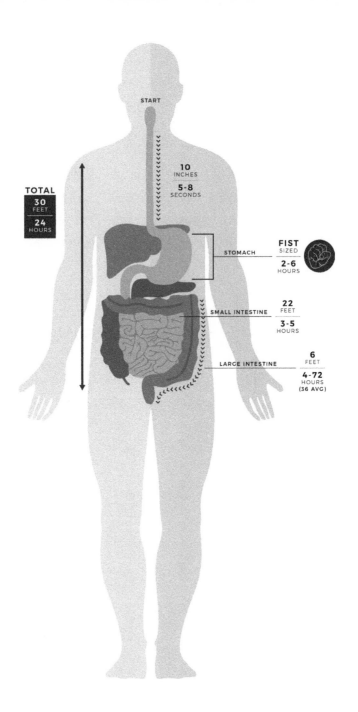

START

TOTAL
30 FEET
24 HOURS

10 INCHES
5-8 SECONDS

STOMACH
FIST SIZED
2-6 HOURS

SMALL INTESTINE
22 FEET
3-5 HOURS

LARGE INTESTINE
6 FEET
4-72 HOURS
(36 AVG)

SARAH

Sarah is starting to get past her time objections. Recently, she realized she's been doing meals all wrong. Her focus has been on feeding her kids—first spoon-feeding one in a high chair, and then making other things for the older ones. As a result, she doesn't eat with her kids and is starving by the time she puts them to bed.

Even during the day, she doesn't take time for her own nutrition needs. When she does eat, she's ashamed of her choices, hiding in the bathroom to eat a candy bar so her kids don't see her. Invariably, they start knocking on the door. "What's that crinkly sound in there?"

"Nothing, go away!" she says.

Finally, a light bulb goes off in her head. This isn't the kind of choice a healthy person makes! Since that realization, she has decided to start modeling good eating habits for her kids. It's not easy at first; her kids have never seen her taking care of herself. They never see Mommy eat. Plus, adjusting mealtimes and expectations has proven a little tricky.

However, Sarah remembers her *real why* and her SMARTER Goals, so she throws herself into the effort. Every meal, she now sits down to eat with her kids, chewing slowly, enjoying her food, and stopping and leaving something on her plate. These are the things she wants her kids to learn, and they'll learn a lot more from seeing her do it.

Apart from the baby food, there are no separate menus. If mommy is eating broccoli, everyone is eating broccoli. Nothing is perfect—sometimes chicken tenders and mac and cheese find their way onto the plate—but Sarah is already seeing her children behave and regard their mommy differently. It's a good start, and soon Sarah will be ready to try more advanced eating habits.

FINAL FOOD THOUGHTS

I could write a whole book on healthy eating. A lot of other people already have. In one chapter, I can only show you the tip of the iceberg. Before you go, though, here are a few more things to help you get going.

OTHER RESOURCES

The interwebs have plenty of great information for you if you know where to look. Here are a few places to go to help reinforce your new healthy eating habits:

- **The Official Habit That Website** (www.drhope-health.com). I'm growing the website and will keep adding content, such as healthy eating ideas and goal setting. Also, don't forget to join the community of other healthy-minded people on the Habit That Tribe Facebook page.

- **The World's Healthiest Foods** (http://whfoods.com). Want some healthy food ideas while boning up on random food trivia? This site offers plenty of learning opportunities. If you want to know all about bananas, here you'll learn their origin, the proper conditions for growth, and proper storage and handling.
- **NutritionFacts.org.** This site is free of lobbying and commercial bias about foods and food groups. The site sells no supplements and accepts no bribes.
- **The Mayo Clinic.** A great evidence-based site for health information. Well-known for their excellent care, the Mayo team has online information about healthy eating habits and more!
- **The Centers for Disease Control and Prevention.** A great place to get facts about diseases, statistics, and disease prevention.

The more you learn, the more you'll feel empowered. However, as my next parting tip explains, there is a caveat.

WATCH OUT FOR FADS

A very smart friend of mine keeps falling for gimmicky fad diets. A while back, he told me he couldn't eat beans.

When I asked why, he said, "Cause I heard there's lectins in beans."

"Okay, what's the bad part about that?" I asked, genuinely curious.

"I don't know," he replied, "but there was a whole book about it, so now I can't eat beans."

More recently, he decided to go on a food cleanse, which has been super popular the past few years. Never mind that your body naturally detoxes and most of those approaches are based on pseudo-science. I don't want to digress too far into a rant, but let's just say that when someone says "toxins," I assume they're going to follow that word up with a whole bunch of BS.

Here's the bottom line. If a diet has a funky name, encourages strange portioning, or tells you to eat extra bacon, it's probably wrong.

Give something the common sense test before you get on the bandwagon. As my dad likes to say, "It's important to have a keen grasp of the obvious."

Granted, sometimes the obvious *can* be hard to grasp with all the different food-related marketing messages floating around. Advertisers will have you believing all kinds of stuff—like that rice cakes are a diet food, milk is the only way to grow strong bones, and bananas are a miracle food and the world's only source of potassium.

Any of those foods can be fine, but it's all about context and nutritional value. A banana a day is great, but four or five is pushing it with all that sugar.

FOOD SHOULD BE REAL

Speaking of sugar, you've probably heard this before, but avoid high-fructose corn syrup whenever you can. It's not a real food. Our bodies don't process it the same way we process natural sugar, and it's been strongly linked to obesity. I don't recommend actively seeking out sugars anyway, since you'll get them naturally as part of a healthy diet, but if you're going for something sugary, make it real.

This goes for everything you eat. You shouldn't have to read complex labels on a box. My kids eat things called apples, broccoli, turkey, and salmon. We live by the rot rule. If it doesn't rot, or if it has a ton of ingredients, then it's not a real food. You are what you eat.

My dad and I had a carton of ice cream once, and we accidentally left it in the sink overnight. We came back the next morning, and it hadn't melted. We were both horrified. What had we put in our bodies?

From then on, we made a rule: if we were going to eat ice cream, it would be from a brand that used sugar, cream, and cookies—no BS fake chemical food. Your body doesn't recognize fake ingredients. It understands vegetables and fruit. Feed your body what it knows.

SARAH'S TOP TEN HEALTHY EATING LIST

To help her make good choices (and to model them for her kids), Sarah has come up with a top ten list of healthy eating practices. She's found they're perfect for her busy life and easy to remember. (Hint: you can use these ideas for your own five-minute health-ups!)

#1. CREATE CONVENIENCE FOODS

Chop up your veggies and portion them in to-go containers so they're ready to grab the next morning. Sarah isn't much of a morning person, so especially on nights before an early shift, she preps the next day's breakfast, lunch, and even snacks like veggies, protein bars, and mixed nuts. By doing this, Sarah is becoming a master of creating convenience foods.

Sarah has heard that it's better to chop up food right before you eat it so it's fresher and has more nutrients. This *is* true, but she also understands that not-quite-as-fresh veggies are still better than no veggies at all.

It may not be the most perfect of all perfect practices, but creating convenience foods is time-effective and health-forward.

#2. PLAN YOUR MEALS IN ADVANCE

Sarah and her family enjoy Taco Tuesday every week. Knowing that allows her to plan accordingly. Not only do they health-up their tacos by adding lettuce and sautéed veggies, they also plan to eat salmon every Wednesday. By removing the choice and planning ahead, it keeps Sarah from making bad decisions. No more Cheetos and candy bar meals in the closet for her!

It's also helped with her shopping and her food prep. Not everything is homemade from scratch—Sarah isn't trying to be Martha Stewart—but she's getting great at supplementing premade foods with healthier ingredients. For instance, she's found that premade quinoa, chopped veggies, or even leafy greens are super healthy add-ins to canned soups.

#3. LOOK AT MENUS BEFORE YOU GO

Historically, Sarah has felt uncomfortable ordering in social settings. When she sees everybody else ordering some big greasy menu item, her impulse is to order something similar, even though that's not what she wants for her body. Because she's felt a little more empowered lately, however, Sarah sticks to her guns today.

"Oh. You're being so healthy," one friend says.

"Oh, now you're making me feel bad about my burger," another says.

Sarah isn't sure how to reply. She doesn't want to make anyone uncomfortable, but she also doesn't think her own choices should matter to anyone else.

She's learned to deflect the comments. "You know, I have stuff to do later and don't want to feel tired," she might say, or simply, "This is just what sounded good." Then she changes the conversation to something else.

It's too bad that guilt and shame can follow us to social situations—increasing the likelihood of an impulsive decision that isn't aligned with our health plans. After almost catching herself ordering a greasy burger a few too many times, Sarah has created a little checkpoint for herself. Now she looks ahead at online menus so she has a plan. This way, she knows exactly what she wants and makes it a point to be the first to order so that others' orders don't tempt her.

#4. BRING THE HEALTHY DISH TO THE POTLUCK

There's always plenty to eat at a get-together, but lately Sarah has been aware that most spreads could use a couple more healthy options. She's decided to become the person who brings a healthy dish—even if she's the only one who eats it.

For those moments when bringing a healthy dish simply isn't an option, Sarah chooses to eat something healthy ahead of time. That way, she's not starving when she gets to the event, she can better limit her food and portion choices, and she can enjoy herself, grazing lightly on the unhealthy stuff.

#5. TAKE ADVANTAGE OF MINDFUL AND MINDLESS EATING

If someone gives you a Hershey's Kiss, what do you do? Most likely, you take it, quickly unwrap it, pop it in your mouth, swallow it, and then find yourself wanting another one.

Sarah has been thinking a lot about this lately. As an experiment, she's been trying to see how long she can stretch the pleasure out of even one little Kiss. Now, she unwraps the chocolate, smells it, and takes little bites. It reveals a whole experience that she'd usually just bypassed. Afterward, she's enjoyed herself so much that she's not especially interested in another Kiss.

Food is many things. It's social, sensual, and attached to a variety of experiences. We use all our senses to enjoy food—smell, taste, touch, sight, and even sound. Sarah doesn't want to mindlessly eat the foods she enjoys. She wants to experience them with every sense.

Naturally, Sarah still wants to graze mindlessly from time to time. That's where chopping her veggies ahead of time has come in handy. Now, Sarah always has a convenient, but healthy, mindless option, which allows her to be mindful, take her time, and enjoy her favorite sweets later.

#6. IF YOU LIKE IT, EAT IT SLOW. IF YOU DON'T LIKE IT, EAT IT FAST.

Sarah's husband has an interesting quirk. He eats the thing he likes the least on his dinner plate first—and really quickly—and then he slows down to enjoy the rest of his meal. Sarah is teaching her kids that, too. Otherwise, they hold off on the vegetables until the end and eat them slowly, especially if it's not their favorite. Sarah's new motto is, "Eat it first, then you have the rest of the meal to enjoy all the things you like!"

#7. SPICE UP YOUR LIFE

Spices have high antioxidant and anti-inflammatory components. It's like adding a little antioxidant, anticancer punch to your meals. There's almost no downside. Plus, they make food less boring.

Experimenting with spices has been an unexpected, fun component of Sarah's new healthy eating goals. She hits the markets for interesting dried and fresh spices and puts them on everything. It's fun and it's healthy.

Before this, Sarah had spices in her cabinet from 1982—and she was a kid in 1982, so she's not sure how she got them. Now, Sarah has turned over everything in her spice rack and filled it with things like basil, oregano, thyme, sage, rosemary, and cinnamon.

She has even created fun games with her kids. She will pull out a few spices at a meal, have them close their eyes and smell them to guess what they are. This helps familiarize them with new flavors and reduce the likelihood they'll start hollering when suspicious specks appear on their food.

#8. ADD VEGETABLES TO ANYTHING, EVEN
PREPACKAGED FOOD

Sarah has begun experimenting with her kids. Recently, she snuck some black beans into her brownies without telling them—and they loved it. It's an easy thing to add to her brownie mix and a nice compromise between homemade and premade. Plus, little touches like this make it a whole lot easier to check off those weekly food boxes.

#9. COOKING OR TOPPING VEGGIES IS FINE!

If you need to put toppings on your vegetables or quinoa to make it palatable, go for it. Eventually, you'll probably find that your taste buds will change and you won't need them anymore.

This goes for microwaving, too. Sarah read that it's not great to microwave vegetables, but again, she also knows that microwaved vegetables are better than *no* vegetables. A little Parmesan cheese on her broccoli is better than no broccoli at all.

After a few weeks of this, Sarah notices herself dialing down these toppings anyway. Plus, now that she's eating more fresh foods, she's noticed herself much more sensitive to the salt and artificial flavors in prepackaged foods.

#10. PORTION FOOD IN ADVANCE

Sarah now makes conscious decisions when she's going to eat and enjoy something. If she's going to eat a piece of cake, she does exactly that—and she doesn't hide in the bathroom from her kids when she does it. Instead, she portions the cake out, looks at it, and says, "Yes, this

is a portion that I'm comfortable with." Then she enjoys
the hell out of it.

CHAPTER 5

SLEEP

When I was pregnant, I was very sick, and as a result my daughter was born underweight.[12] My pediatrician and I set a goal for me to try to nurse her every two hours to get her up to an appropriate weight.

The nights were the hardest. In order to help me out, my husband would get up, change our daughter, and bring her to me so I could have an extra few minutes of sleep.

---

12 Here's a little beginning-of-the-chapter mini nerd alert: my condition during pregnancy, *hyperemesis gravidarium*, is more than morning sickness. It is a severe form of persistent vomiting. Princess Kate Middleton was afflicted with it as well—though she still managed to look like a beautiful princess, whereas I looked slightly better than death warmed over and with unkempt hair. I had a PICC line (a special long-term IV) for both of my pregnancies, and was so sick with the second one that I had a feeding tube from my nose to my intestines to provide nutrition. Speaking of, here's another interesting fact I learned: you can throw up around a feeding tube. It was unpleasant. Fortunately, this condition is rare. And despite my fears and other complications, both of my kids turned out just fine. They are healthy, happy, active, adorable little maniacs, and I am eternally grateful!

One time, he brought her to me like usual—except this time, after handing our daughter off, he just stood there staring at me.

Exhausted to the max and not in the friendliest mood, I said, "What? Why are you staring at me?"

"Would you like the baby?" he asked.

"I already have the baby!" I snapped.

"You're nursing a stuffed giraffe."

I was about to make some other smartass retort, but then I realized he may have a point. My daughter wasn't latching very well—and she was way fuzzier than normal.

"Oh, yeah," I said, trying to laugh it off. "That's a giraffe pillow pet. I see that now. Okay, hand me the baby."

Instead, he said, "Nope, we're good here," and then he backed away and gave her a bottle instead.

I collapsed back into my pillow and didn't wake up again for several hours.

WE'VE ALL BEEN SLEEP-DEPRIVED

The giraffe incident wasn't the only time I've been sleep-deprived. Aside from the many sleepless nights that come with having two kids, there were also the eighty-hour-plus workweeks I used to put in during the residency phase of my medical training—and the twenty-four-hour shifts I still work up to a few times a month for my side job at a rural critical-access hospital.

During these marathon shifts, I'm sometimes lucky if I can get a few hours of uninterrupted sleep. There is no way to plan, patients come when they come, and I'm responsible for taking care of whomever walks through the door, regardless of the time of day or night. So, naturally, I'm pretty wiped out by the time I have to make the two-hour drive home when I'm done!

Although I love the work and the people, for the sake of my sleep, I try not to work too many of these shifts a month. While I certainly feel good providing much-needed medical care to rural communities, the reality is that sleep deprivation isn't good for anyone, especially doctors. In fact, going without sleep for long enough can literally kill you.

Before you panic, don't worry. You have to go a long time before this happens. How long, exactly, science still isn't sure. But eventually, the chemical changes resulting from sleep deprivation cause something else to go wrong. Maybe you'll have a heart attack. Maybe you'll get in a car wreck. Maybe you'll snap and commit suicide. Bleak stuff, I know, but sleep deprivation has been a driving factor in all these unfortunate outcomes.

The *Guinness Book of World Records* used to have a record for the most consecutive days of staying awake. But after seeing how dangerous sleep deprivation actually was, they removed all prior records and wisely refused to indulge any further record-breaking attempts.

WHAT HAPPENS WHEN YOU DON'T SLEEP

Perhaps you've had a moment in your life when you were exercising and eating well—you were doing everything right, dammit—and still you weren't seeing the results you expected. If you ignore the sleep pillar and only allow yourself a few hours of crappy sleep a night, it doesn't matter what you do elsewhere. Sleep deprivation puts your body into full-on fight-or-flight mode. And when your body is trying to survive, it doesn't care about how great your abs look. It's only interested in trying to stay alive.

BAD BODY CHEMISTRY

When you go into fight-or-flight mode, a lot of bad things happen. Your adrenaline jacks up, making you feel anxious, wired, and tense. You may want to go to sleep, but because you've been sending your body so many mixed signals, it doesn't believe you. It's hoarding energy and trying to keep you alive, making weight loss out of the question. You feel tired and wired; it is not a good state to be in.

In fact, because lack of sleep leads to increased insulin levels, you're more likely to gain weight. Also, everything hurts because your nerves are more sensitive and have fewer opportunities to repair themselves. The same thing happens to your immune system, which means you're not only walking around feeling exhausted, but you're also vulnerable to every cold going around.

Your testosterone and libido drop, too, which is no fun for anyone. Plus, the extra cortisol your body is producing breaks down the collagen in your skin, makes you more wrinkly, and gives you puffy, dark circles around your eyes. Yep, that's right. When you're chronically sleep-deprived, you look older and less attractive.

Have you ever started craving greasy food when you're up past your bedtime? That's your body saying, "If you won't give me sleep, you need to give me some kind of crappy fuel in order to combat this crappy schedule." It's easy to make bad choices when your body keeps egging you on like that. I don't blame you for wanting to give in.

BYE-BYE COPING SKILLS

When you're not getting enough sleep, your coping skills go down. If you have kids, you've seen the symptoms. On days that they miss their naps, they lose their minds over the smallest stuff. When they're well-rested, though, they're nice, normal, well-adjusted little humans. Sure, if your kids are anything like mine when they're well-rested, they're also high-energy ninja maniac whirlwinds—but at least they're in a good mood as they tear through the house.

We often don't think of children in terms of sleep deprivation. However, studies have shown that children who are diagnosed with ADD or ADHD often aren't getting enough sleep. The vast majority of these sleep-deprived kids experience worse school performance, worse concentration, and worse behavior.

This extends all the way to the upper levels of school. High schools with an early start time see impaired performance on test scores—whether the subject is reading, math, or science. When they shift high school start times to later in the morning and make no other additional changes in curriculum, test scores go up.[13]

---

13   To learn more about the relationship between school start times and student performance, start here: Robert Marx, Emily E. Tanner-Smith, Colleen M Davison, Lee-Anne Ufholz, John Freeman, Ravi Shankar, Lisa Newton, Robert S. Brown, Alyssa S. Parpia, Ioana Cozma, and Shawn Hendrikx, "Later School Start Times for Supporting the Education, Health and Well-Being of High School Students," Campbell Collaboration, December 19, 2017, https://www.campbellcollaboration.org/library/later-school-start-times-education-health-well-being-high-school-students.html.

Parents have a big role in this. They often put their kids to bed too late and wake them up too early, all but guaranteeing inadequate sleep. To be fair, sometimes these challenges are tied to economics. If mommy or daddy has to be at work by six, they have to wake their kids up by five to get them to day care. In this situation, the only real way to combat this kind of sleep deprivation is through an earlier bedtime.[14]

NERD ALERT: THE SIGNS OF SLEEP DEPRIVATION

Want a good, easy-to-reference laundry list of sleep deprivation symptoms? I've got just the thing! Chronic lack of sleep can lead to:

- Memory problems
- Depression
- Impaired concentration
- Higher ghrelin levels, which leads to more cravings for high-fat and sugary foods (cheap, easy fuel)
- Higher insulin, which leads to more weight gain
- Impaired immune function, leading you to catch every cold you come across
- Increased perception of pain

14 Multiple studies back up the effect of sleep, or sleep deprivation, on childhood development. For a good overview, I recommend this article from the National Sleep Foundation: https://sleepfoundation.org/sleep-news/backgrounder-later-school-start-times.

- Decreased coping skills
- Lower libido
- Lower testosterone
- Increased adrenaline
- Difficulty with memory consolidation
- Worse mood
- Increased chance of diabetes
- Wrinkled skin (increased cortisol production breaks down collagen)
- Premature death
- Microsleeps
- Delirium and hallucinations
- Impaired task performance
- Impaired coordination
- Significant hormonal changes
- Impaired judgment and decision-making (similar to drunk shopping on Amazon)

BASICALLY, YOU'RE DRUNK

The consequence of sleep deprivation over even twenty-four hours is comparable to the cognitive impairment of someone with a 0.1 blood alcohol level. That means if you're driving around ultra-tired, you're basically driving around drunk.

Unfortunately, this impairment extends far beyond driving. It impacts every function—working, parenting, exercising, you name it. Nobody would think it was acceptable to come to work drunk, and yet we high-five the workaholics who pull all-nighters.

We haven't even talked about decision-making yet. Have you ever been drunk and up late shopping on Amazon? There's an entire hashtag dedicated to the funny things people bought online when they were drunk.[15] We don't make great decisions when we're drunk, and we don't make great decisions when we're sleep-deprived, either. As Alcoholics Anonymous likes to say, "Don't ever make big decisions when you are HALT: hungry, angry, lonely, tired," because you make terrible decisions in these states.

I think about this all the time at my job, where many days bring life-or-death decisions. I owe it to my patients not to be tired. You may not have to worry about sticking a tube down somebody's trachea to put them on life support, but you probably do have to worry about making big financial decisions, managing your relationships, or even deciding what kind of car to buy. Do you want to be doing this when you're functionally impaired?

SLEEP DEPRIVATION IS NOT A BADGE OF HONOR

You can't make up for lost sleep easily. When I work those

---

15 For some laughs, check out the hashtag #drunkamazonshopping on Twitter, Instagram, or the like. A quick Google search will also turn up some great articles on the subject.

twenty-four-hour shifts, I may not have gotten much useful sleep, but I still have to function for my family once I get home. I don't usually feel fully rested again for several days. It's not something I like doing, but I've accepted that sometimes it's part of the job.

Some people wear sleep deprivation like a badge of honor. I've even heard surgeons say things like, "Oh, I can burn a candle on both ends during the week and then just sleep twelve hours on Friday and Saturday to make up for it." But it doesn't work like that. That extra sleep on the weekend might feel good, but without a balanced sleep cycle, you're still doing your body more harm than good.

People often hide behind work as the reason they can't sleep. The thing is, the longer you go without useful sleep, the more you impair your work performance, and the less you accomplish. You'll actually be more productive if you stop what you are doing and get a good night's rest.

As a society, we need to stop high-fiving people for walking around like drunken bad-decision-makers. We need to recognize and reward healthy behavior. You can start by recognizing and rewarding yourself!

NERD ALERT: THE LATE-NIGHT EXAM CRAM

Are you one of those people who pulls all-nighters cramming for exams or knocking out big work projects? If so, you should know you're not doing yourself any favors.

In one study, three groups of participants were taught something complex. Afterward, the first group was sent home for a regular night's sleep, the second was deliberately sleep-deprived for the night, and the third group slept normally for one night but was sleep-deprived the next night. Three days later, among all the participants, the second and third groups had a considerably more difficult time accurately remembering what they had been taught.

In other words, it may feel like you're helping yourself out with those late-nights study sessions, but in reality, you're not learning in a meaningful way. The best thing you can do is get a good night's sleep. This will substantially consolidate your memory—one of your body's main tasks while you're zonked out.[16]

---

16 If you want to read up on more of this, I recommend the following resources: Mark Wheeler, "Cramming for a Test? Don't Do It, Say UCLA Researchers," UCLA Newsroom, August 22, 2012, http://newsroom.ucla.edu/releases/cramming-for-a-test-don-t-do-it-237733; Amy Reichelt, "Revising for Exams—Why Cramming the Night Before Rarely Works," The Conversation, October 27, 2016, http://theconversation.com/revising-for-exams-why-cramming-the-night-before-rarely-works-67459; and "Sleep Deprivation and Memory Loss," WebMD, 2018, https://www.webmd.com/sleep-disorders/sleep-deprivation-effects-on-memory#1.

THE CAFFEINE CYCLE

"I added a tenth cup of coffee to my day. Now I can see noises!"

When you don't get a good night's sleep, you crave stimulants like coffee. To be fair, it's okay to enjoy a cup or two of coffee at the right time of day, but if you're drinking a pot at night within a few hours of bedtime (something I know plenty of people do), you're depriving your body of the deep, restorative sleep you need. When you're caffeinated, your sleep is lighter and more easily interruptible, and you wake up the next morning feeling tired.

Of course, the more tired you feel in the morning, the more coffee you feel the need to drink. Meanwhile, your body is pumping out all this adrenaline to help keep you awake. You may be exhausted, but after even a few nights on this kind of caffeine cycle, you'll find yourself lying in bed, wide awake, unable to sleep because of all the caffeine and adrenaline pumping through your veins. You'll wake up exhausted once again, and then you'll repeat the cycle.

Soon, the caffeine isn't enough to get you going, and all that adrenaline isn't helping much anymore, either. This calls for more drastic measures, so you decide to take a sleeping pill or start having a few drinks before bed, mistakenly assuming those things will help you sleep.

The problem is, the sleeping pill will impair higher-level

functions and disrupt your sleep cycle. And while alcohol does make you a bit sleepy, it also likes to wake you up in the middle of the night on its way out of your system. In other words, you may have been able to fall asleep better, but you never reached a deep level of sleep, and that early morning wakeup just sets you further behind.

I know a lot of people who say they can't sleep without some kind of pill. They try to wean off of sleep aids for a night or two, but they're wired at three in the morning and telling themselves it's useless. Since your brain believes what you say, it goes along with you and lets you stay awake.

Prescription sleep aids rank among the most prescribed medications in the country.[17] Getting off the caffeine-to-sleep-aid cycle is as hard as quitting smoking or detoxing off a drug, which is why so many people can't escape it. I'm not anti-caffeine, but I only support it in a limited, only-before-noon basis.

BUT WAIT, I HEARD COFFEE IS GOOD!

If you make, sell, or just plain enjoy coffee, you're more likely to believe that coffee is purely good for you and has no bad side effects. It's easy to find articles that support this perspective, and they're not totally wrong. Coffee

---

17   As of this writing, Ambien is number twelve on the list.

does have antioxidants and other beneficial properties as long as you're not spiking it with a bunch of sugar and chemicals.

There are other health benefits to coffee, too. Caffeine can improve your work performance. It can improve your cognition at the appropriate dose, and it can even improve athletic performance.

However, caffeine also interferes with sleep. Period. You have to balance out the good and the bad. If you want to maximize the benefits of coffee and minimize the drawbacks, drink it early in the day.

This will be a challenge for those of you who rely on caffeine to get out of those midafternoon slumps. (Remember the hangry moments we talked about last chapter?) It's too late in the day for a stimulant, though, even if you think you've built up a tolerance.

While we're on the subject, the whole idea of tolerance is misleading. Let's compare it to alcohol. You probably know (or knew in college) someone who's very proud they can drink a dozen beers without feeling drunk. However, just because that person doesn't feel trashed doesn't mean those twelve beers aren't wreaking havoc on their system.

It's the same thing with caffeine. You may feel fine after

two pots of coffee, but it's still in there stimulating your adrenaline and triggering other chemical processes. Just because you're a bit desensitized to it doesn't mean it's not impairing your ability to get a good night's sleep.

WEAN THE CAFFEINE

Caffeine is a drug. When you try to quit it, you go into withdrawal. One or two servings is fine, but if you're getting more than this—especially at night—perhaps a SMARTER Goal would be to taper your intake down to the recommended amount.

Also, I'm sorry to say this, but no energy drinks. They're only a small step above poison (and they taste like a combination of medicine and awfulness!). With their fake sugars and other crash-inducing ingredients, they wreak havoc on your insulin and digestive cycles and are chock-full of pro-inflammatory chemicals.

It's not glamorous, but my recommendation is plain coffee and tea—decaf, preferably. If you want to relax in the evenings, a warm cup of herbal tea is great before bedtime.

All this connects with a lot of things we talked about last chapter. Generally speaking, you don't want to drink your calories, especially with the out-of-control portions we're used to seeing. One time, I was in the car with my aunt, who stopped at a Starbucks drive-through and ordered a quad-shot of espresso in the largest-sized cup. The person on the other end of the drive-through laughed and said, "You must be having a rough day!" If your coffee orders are making even your baristas blush, you probably need to dial it down.

To be totally clear, if you love coffee, I'm not suggesting cutting it out completely. Part of being a healthy person is having fun. I don't want you miserable and mad at me because I told you to quit one of your favorite things. However, I am recommending that you limit your intake and stick to drinking it only in the mornings.

NERD ALERT: DOWN WITH ENERGY DRINKS!

The alarming amount of caffeine in energy drinks isn't the only problem. As we've discussed, caffeine has its good and bad points; the more you consume and the later in the day you consume it, the worse off you are. The problem with so-called energy drinks is that, in addition to all that caffeine, you're loading up on a whole bunch of sugar and a chemical soup of crap designed to stimulate your body. To top it off, all the extra vitamins, taurine, guarana, and other herbals they throw in are in higher concentrations than we would get in food. Combine everything together, and we end up overstimulating our bodies in a potentially dangerous way.

Here's a short list of known complications from drinking can after can of this crap:

- Cardiac arrest (Yes, death. That will definitely not improve your energy or performance!)
- Headaches
- Nausea and vomiting
- Elevated blood pressure
- Seizures
- Increased anxiety
- Jitteriness and nervousness
- Insomnia
- Addiction
- Risky behavior or "Toxic Jock Syndrome"[18]
- Interactions with medications and supplements

Here's the bottom line: step away from the pumped-up hype and get your energy from nutritious food, energizing exercise, restorative rest, and releasing stress. It will be easier on your tongue (seriously, these drinks taste like ass), your body, and your wallet.

HERE'S HOW YOU HABIT THAT

Once you start to understand what both a lack of sleep and

---

18 New York Times News Service, "Toxic Jock Syndrome," *Chicago Tribune*, May 28, 2008, http://articles.chicagotribune.com/2008-05-28/news/0805280578_1_energy-drinks-spike-shooter-red-bull.

regular sleep can do to you, it's a lot easier to start creating better habits and get your body back into a natural cycle. Here are my favorite sleep hygiene recommendations.

EVERYONE'S SLEEP NEEDS ARE DIFFERENT

Different ages require slightly different amounts of sleep time. Kids need anywhere from fourteen to sixteen hours when they're little, though that number gradually decreases as they get older. Most adults should be getting between seven and nine hours of sleep, with seven being the bare minimum for good restorative sleep.

I have friends who love to say they can get by fine on only a few hours of sleep. I tend to need a little more to feel rested. Similarly, some people are natural morning people, and some are naturally night owls. That's their body chemistry. Even as a toddler, I slept later than most kids, while my brother, at the same age, was bright, sunny, and wide awake at five o'clock—even on Christmas morning! Don't get me wrong, I was a big fan of Christmas, too, but, as I liked to remind my brother, the presents could wait. No one was going to swoop in and steal them while we slept in.

Whatever the case, there's a big difference between getting by and being optimal, and we need to plan our sleep cycles accordingly. I may be a night owl, but I also have to get my eight or nine hours of sleep. I can't be up working until two in the morning if I have to be up at seven the next day.

If you're living with someone whose sleep needs are different than yours, sleeping arrangements can be tricky. After all, you don't want to wake your spouse up when you come to bed in the middle of the night, and they probably don't want to wake you up at five in the morning when they wake up. The first thing to do is see if you can compromise on a sleep schedule that suits both of you. If not, I've known some couples who choose to sleep separately sometimes, just so they can get some rest.

KEEP A ROUTINE

The modern sleep cycle is less than ideal:

Sleep late → wake up tired → promise to sleep early → the internet → repeat

That said, turning things around doesn't have to be a chore. The best sleep scientists recommend that you go to sleep and get up at the same time every day. On weekends, we tend to stay up late, sleep in late, and try to binge on sleep (and Netflix), but it's not doing us much good. You can't bank sleep.

Every night, try to give yourself a minimum eight-hour sleep opportunity, meaning that you're in bed eight hours before your alarm goes off. To be clear, I mean a full, uninterrupted eight hours with the lights off. And make sure you're only counting the time when you're actually *in* bed—brushing your teeth and checking your phone don't count! You may not get a full eight hours of sleep since falling asleep takes time, but at least you're allowing yourself that much time to rest.

If you get up consistently at the same time every day, your body internalizes this schedule, minimizing the need for an alarm. In fact, if you need an alarm or if you're still groggy when you wake up, then you're probably not going to bed early enough. That's the trickiest part for some people. My advice? Set an alarm to tell you when to go to bed, not just when to wake up.

Another good thing about finding a routine is it helps you wake up at the right point in your sleep cycle. Have you ever been dead asleep and then rudely awakened, causing you to feel like crap the rest of the day? Most likely, it's because you woke up at the wrong time in your sleep cycle and ruined your dream about being a unicorn-riding ninja fighting zombie pirates. If this happens to you consistently, you're walking around functionally impaired every day. The best way to counteract this is simple: go to bed earlier.

COOL, DARK, AND QUIET

"I just had a fight with my alarm clock. It wanted me to get up. I disagreed. Things got violent. Now it's broken and I'm wide awake. Not sure which of us won."

Biologically, our body temperature is supposed to drop along with the outside temperature. That's our body's signal to go to sleep. Although modern heating is a godsend if you live somewhere like my home state of Michigan, it's screwing with our sleep cycles.

We need cool, dark, and quiet for good sleep hygiene. The ideal sleeping temperature is cooler than you might think. Generally, you want to shoot for a range between sixty and sixty-seven degrees. If you've got a programmable thermostat, this is an easy fix to make.

Another way to kick your body into sleep mode is by taking a warm shower. When you step out, the cooler air triggers your body temperature to start dropping. This is also a great way to relax and wash off the day's worries and signal to your body and mind that you've done all you can for the day—which makes it a great five-minute health-up for daily stress management (see Chapter 7). I consider this calm, relaxing time an essential part of my nighttime routine, something I look forward to and reward myself with every day.

To give yourself dark and quiet, the best thing you can do is ban electronics from your bedroom. I like to say that your bedroom should be for nothing but sleep and sex. You shouldn't be watching TV or fiddling with your smartphone in the bedroom—so keep them out! It's nice that your phone has an alarm feature, but it also has a lot of other features that distract you and disturb your circadian rhythms. Best to just invest four bucks in a plug-in alarm and get a better night's sleep.

WHAT IF YOU CAN'T SLEEP?

If you're a human being, and I'm pretty sure you are, you've probably had nights when you just couldn't fall asleep. That happens to all of us.

Unfortunately, I see a lot of bad advice out there on how to deal with restlessness at night. A lot of people recommend watching TV or reading books, but both of those activities expose your brain to light and stimulation—pretty much the opposite of what you need to fall asleep.

Falling asleep watching TV might sound harmless, but even after you're asleep, that blue light is messing with you, and all that noise is keeping you from reaching the deepest levels of sleep. If you're going to read, read a physical book or magazine in dim, yellow non-full-spectrum lighting. Smartphone or tablet screens are simply too stimulating.

What do you do instead? There's no one perfect option. Some nights, you just have to accept it. That said, I'll share some things I've tried. For starters, I turn the clock away from me so I'm not fixating on what time it is. As a healthy person, instead of stressing about being awake, I congratulate myself for giving my body and my brain an opportunity to rest in a cool, dark place.

From there, I might try some brain exercises and allow myself to daydream. (Yes, you can daydream at night in bed.) I let this daydream out-compete other stressful thoughts, which eventually helps my mind to relax. This isn't that different from counting sheep or meditating, but for me, those specific exercises let other thoughts come in.

Judge me all you want, but I'm going to share one of my go-to daydreams when I can't sleep. In it, I am a superhero who can teleport and fly, and I have super strength to boot—and perfect hair and an amazing superhero costume, obviously! I get to save people in distress and rid the world of bad guys. Sound silly? With the incredible popularity of superhero movies, I'm betting I'm not the only closet crimefighter wannabe. Plus, it's my dreams, my rules. I get to determine the "reality." I see some sad things in my job as an emergency medicine doctor, and it is fun to have control in a chaotic world sometimes, even if it's a world of my own design.

The cool thing is, you can design your own world, too! It is a form of meditation that is vivid enough to keep other thoughts (about your huge to-do list, your worries, etc.) from creeping in. And it gives you something to look forward to when lying down at night. Eventually, the daydream gives way to sleep, and the fun fantasy world is now a trigger for my brain to relax and let go for the night.

The bottom line is, if your brain's not shutting off right away, it's okay. The rest opportunity is still helpful. It will still put you in a better position for tomorrow than you would be after binge-watching your favorite Netflix show all night. So let yourself go with a nice nighttime daydream. Give yourself the power to do something you've always wanted to do, like fly a plane. The way I see it, most of us rarely get to daydream anyway, and who doesn't like to daydream?

NERD ALERT: THE POWER OF POWER NAPS

As I was writing this book, I saw these articles going around telling people to drink a coffee and then take a twenty- to forty-minute power nap. By the time you wake up, they say, the caffeine is in your system, and you should be raring to go. I find the whole idea fascinating.

In and of themselves, naps can be potentially beneficial. It's no surprise that most societies used to (and some lucky ones still do) have a form of *siesta* in the middle of the day, when the body naturally feels sleepy. All of our bodies feel some form of slump in the early afternoon, and naps in certain situations are great. However, in the modern age, most of our jobs aren't compatible with the *siesta* lifestyle, so our impulse is to load up on sugar and stimulants to keep us going. Here's my advice if your body is screaming for a *siesta* and you can't give it what it wants: get active. Take a walk out in the sun, do some chores, or run up and down the stairs at your office. Give yourself a safe and natural boost of energy and adrenaline without the sugar and caffeine crash from drinks of dubious ingredients.

If none of that works and a nap is the only thing that will get you through the rest of the day, just remember that naps aren't a substitute for sleep. If you need to nap regularly, that's your body telling you that you're not getting enough sleep at night. Further, the later in the day you take a nap, the more you interfere with your normal sleep cycle. People who doze off in front of the TV after dinner, for instance, are usually wide awake at bedtime and can't get back to sleep. Nothing about this behavior is healthy.

If you're going to take a nap, avoid the gimmicky coffee-and-power-doze shenanigans and simply allow yourself an opportunity to rest. Further, make sure you do all your napping before about three o'clock so you don't interfere with your nighttime sleep cycle.

WHY SLEEP IS SO GREAT

What if I could give you a pill that made your brain and organs function better; that improved mood and coordination; that reduced risk of depression, anxiety, heart disease, ADD, and ADHD; that made you look better; and that improved muscle tone and libido? What if I promised there were no adverse side effects either?

Okay, you're right, there is no pill that does all those things. If there were and I discovered it, I would be a trillionaire riding atop flying unicorns around my own private tropical island. But while there may not be a magic pill that provides all these benefits, you know what does? Sleep.

It's odd the way we treat sleep. Everyone loves doing it, everyone loves the benefits it provides, and yet we continually deprive ourselves of it. Why? It's not like there's a trophy for not getting enough sleep.

And yet here I am, right in the middle of a big old chapter all about sleep. Since we're on the subject, we might as well take a look at the chemical processes inside your body that make sleep so beneficial.

MELATONIN IS THE BEST

Most people think of melatonin as an over-the-counter sleep aid. Yes, you can buy melatonin, but it's a lot cheaper to just lie down in a cool, dark, and quiet environment, where your body produces melatonin naturally.

Melatonin is a wonderful, natural, anti-inflammatory hormone whose primary job is to help you relax and fall asleep. It's like your very own personal sandman, and all you have to do for him to show up is turn off the lights; you don't have to take melatonin supplements if you allow your body to produce higher doses of the hormone naturally. If you let it do its job, your body will give you all the melatonin you need.

HUMAN GROWTH HORMONE IS PRETTY GOOD, TOO

You know what else your body produces lots of while you're sleeping? Human growth hormone (HGH). You've probably heard it mentioned as part of an athletic doping scandal, but just like melatonin, your body should be capable of making all you need.

Human growth hormone has so many natural benefits. It builds muscle, burns fat, decreases fat storage, protects your bones, protects you from heart disease, enhances immunity, improves mood, and protects the pancreas and liver. Oh, and it also increases life-span and is considered by some to be an anti-aging hormone. Doesn't that sound great?

Sure, you could go out and inject your body with it, but that route comes with a lot of potential downsides. That's why HGH supplements come with an FDA black box warning.

I say skip the injections and let your body's natural cycles take over. Your pituitary gland produces and releases HGH five times a day—and the longest and largest pulse is during deep sleep (which means you need to get to deep sleep to get the benefit!). If you don't get enough sleep, you rob your body of its ability to produce this amazingly beneficial hormone.

HGH production also increases during exercise, meaning if you exercise during the day and then get a good night's sleep, you're getting the full benefit and none of the risks. Just remember, to get that big HGH dose at night, you need to go through the full sleep cycle of REM and NREM sleep—and you only get there if you're nice and relaxed in a cool, dark, and quiet environment.

NERD ALERT: GOT RHYTHM?

You've probably heard about circadian rhythms. So what exactly is happening in your body? Why do you feel wide-awake, warm, and energetic at certain times during the day, and cold, tired, and sleepy during others? Let's nerd out about the beautiful hormonal symphony occurring in your body each day.

Your body cycles through sleep and awake hormones approximately every twenty-four hours. Cortisol, testosterone, growth hormone, melatonin: all of the usual suspects are here. And if you take advantage of the amazing benefits these hormones offer, your health will improve!

Let's start with the morning. Before waking, your melatonin levels have dipped to daytime levels. Your blood pressure goes up, and you start your day. Around 8:30, you are most likely to have a bowel movement (especially if you've had some coffee!). Your testosterone and cortisol levels go up, increasing your energy and alertness.

Heading into the afternoon, your best coordination will come around 2:30, so plan for activities that require your dexterity in this part of the day to best take advantage of your biological rhythms. Your best reaction time is around 3:30 p.m.; bring on the challenges!

Later in the afternoon, your body temperature takes a little dip as your cortisol begins decreasing. This is when you start to get a little tired and reach for sugar or coffee to boost you up! Instead of unhealthy habits, take advantage of knowing your chemistry. Go for a walk, get active, expose yourself to bright light, and let your body give you a natural energy boost for your efforts.

Your cardiovascular efficacy and muscle strength peak around 5:00 p.m. Why not schedule a workout right around this time so you can feel fit and strong? From here, your blood pressure and body temperature start to go up, peaking by around 7:00 p.m.

At around 9:00, your melatonin production starts—if you don't mess it up with bright lights, that is! Your body suppresses bowel movements around 10:30 p.m. (no one wants to wake up for a nighttime poop!). If you go to sleep when your body wants you to, your deepest sleep will be around 2:00 a.m.

By about 4:30 in the morning, your body temperature will reach its lowest point of the day. If you've ever pulled an all-nighter, you probably remember feeling extra cold right around this time. Even when you force yourself to stay awake, your hormones will continue their cycle—yet another reason that missing sleep is dangerous. When your body is going through all the sleep routines except for sleep itself, you are definitely not in peak performing condition. As the morning progresses, your blood pressure and temperature rise, and the cycle begins again. If you don't screw with Mother Nature, good sleep can be yours!

CIRCADIAN RHYTHMS IN HUMANS

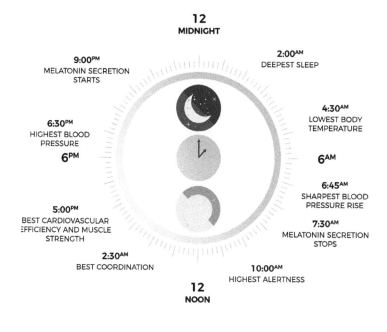

12
MIDNIGHT

9:00ᴾᴹ
MELATONIN SECRETION
STARTS

2:00ᴬᴹ
DEEPEST SLEEP

6:30ᴾᴹ
HIGHEST BLOOD
PRESSURE

4:30ᴬᴹ
LOWEST BODY
TEMPERATURE

6ᴾᴹ

6ᴬᴹ

5:00ᴾᴹ
BEST CARDIOVASCULAR
EFFICIENCY AND MUSCLE
STRENGTH

6:45ᴬᴹ
SHARPEST BLOOD
PRESSURE RISE

7:30ᴬᴹ
MELATONIN SECRETION
STOPS

2:30ᴬᴹ
BEST COORDINATION

10:00ᴬᴹ
HIGHEST ALERTNESS

12
NOON

LOWEST MELATONIN
LEVEL

HIGHEST MELATONIN
LEVEL

WHAT HAPPENS WHEN YOU MISS SLEEP

When you're sleep-deprived, your whole body is screaming at you to lie down and go to sleep. It will even force you asleep if it gets desperate enough. It makes no difference to your body if you're driving, performing a complex surgery, or watching your favorite movie on the couch. Here's what's going on in your body during these sleep-starved moments.

ONE MISSED NIGHT AIN'T SO BAD...IS IT?

If you're generally well-rested and miss one night of good sleep, you'll feel crappy the next day, but you likely won't suffer any significant long-term consequences. However, you can accumulate a sleep debt very quickly, and even one missed night of sleep can lead to memory problems. Start adding up the nights of impaired sleep, and you'll experience weight gain, impaired concentration, memory issues, and increased risk of depression.

In other words, too much missed sleep is serious business—so serious that the Geneva Convention outlawed it as an inhumane torture method.

CLOSED FOR REPAIRS

When you're asleep, your body performs a lot of critical functions it can't do when you're awake. It digests food, heals the body and mind, consolidates memories, and makes sense of experiences, things that are bothering you, and trauma. That's why one of the worst things you can do to a person suffering from PTSD is deprive them of sleep.

I like to pretend that your brain is a big, busy building full of bustling workers, visitors, clients, and delivery people coming and going during the day. At night, the cleaning crew comes in, straightens everything up, cleans up all the mess, and puts everything where it's supposed to be so the next day you're ready to function again. If you don't get to clean up—perhaps because you left the office as a disaster area and only gave your cleaning crew a few minutes to come in and do their job—that mess is still going to be there when you walk into the office, and it's going to affect your work. Your cleaning crew can't do its job unless you give them the chance, just like your body can't repair and ready your brain if you're depriving it of sleep!

If you break your ankle, your doctor is going to tell you to stay off it so it can heal. They're not going to tell you to get up and jump on your ankle every four hours to make sure it's still broken. If your brain has had a rough day—perhaps from overwork or even a more serious injury like a concussion—you need to let it heal in a similar way. Your brain should get *at least* as much respect as your ankle! For any time we need restorative sleep, whether we're sick, stressed, suffering a concussion, or even just at the end of a typical day, doctors recommend brain rest—no TV, no video games, and no phones. Find a cool, dark, relaxing, environment to promote rest and healing.

A TIMELINE OF INCREASED RISK

Poor sleep raises the risk for cancer, heart attack, and stroke because your body has to produce high levels of cortisol, the fight-or-flight hormone, just to keep you running. And because your body isn't able to perform its usual maintenance duties, a lot more fat and plaque ends up getting deposited along your arteries, further increasing your risk.

Sleep deprivation becomes a life-or-death matter remarkably fast. After even thirty-six hours of being awake, the inflammatory markers in your bloodstream have spiked, increasing your risk of cardiovascular disease and high blood pressure. At this point, you're an emotional wreck, the equivalent of a sleep-deprived toddler running around making terrible decisions.

After forty-eight hours of no sleep, your body starts shutting down and throwing you into microsleeps. These can last anywhere from a half-second to a half-minute, each followed by a period of disorientation. That's why driving while sleep deprived is so dangerous. It doesn't matter if you roll down the windows, smack your face, or turn the radio up. Those microsleeps are still going to happen— and they could lead to serious consequences.

Imagine as you're driving home from work late one night, a person is walking innocently along the side of the road. During a brief microsleep, your car drifts just enough to strike the pedestrian. Suddenly, your life has changed forever! Strangely, many people don't worry enough about what might happen to themselves if they fall asleep behind the wheel and crash (which is a whole other problem!). However, please consider the consequences of accidentally taking the life of another.

After seventy-two hours (three full days) of sleep deprivation, you are now a psychotic, drunken, uncoordinated toddler. Even a simple conversation with somebody feels exhausting. Your coordination, motivation, perception, and higher mental processes are fully and obviously impaired, and you can start hallucinating. These hallucinations are no laughing matter, by the way. They can lead to violence and suicidal impulses.

Granted, most of us don't stay up continuously for seventy-two hours. That's pretty hard to relate to. However, if you're only getting three or four hours of sleep at night, all the functional impairments, save for psychosis, are making themselves known. Without question, you are operating at a diminished capacity from your accumulated sleep debt. I don't know about you, but running around like a confused, drunken toddler isn't exactly how I want to spend the rest of my life.

NERD ALERT: WHAT HAPPENS TO YOUR
BODY WHEN YOU DON'T SLEEP?

In 1942, people were averaging 7.9 hours of sleep a night. In 2013, that number had dropped to 6.8 hours.[19] What happened? Why such a big difference? A big contributing factor is that we have a lot more to distract us these days. There's always something to do, and many of us try to do as much as we can. Our bodies, however, still need the same amount of sleep as they always did, otherwise sleep deprivation will start to set in.

Sleep deprivation leads to symptoms similar to drunk driving. According to the National Highway Traffic Safety Administration, driver fatigue is responsible for an estimated 83,000 motor vehicle accidents and about 850 deaths each year. Some researchers, though, believe the numbers are actually much higher.[20]

The longer you go without sleep, the crazier the symptoms become:

- **At twenty-four hours**, your cognitive impairment is equivalent to having a blood alcohol content of 0.10 percent, which is above the legal limit of 0.08 in most states. Your coping skills diminish, your focus diminishes, and your senses dull.

---

19 Jeffrey M. Jones, "In US, 40 Percent Get Less Than Recommended Amount of Sleep," Gallup, December 19, 2013, http://news.gallup.com/poll/166553/less-recommended-amount-sleep.aspx.

20 National Highway Traffic Safety Administration, "Drowsy Driving," https://www.nhtsa.gov/risky-driving/drowsy-driving.

- **At forty-eight hours**, you're highly disoriented, and your body is trying to cope by shutting down for tiny micro-sleeps. Essentially, you're like a toddler whose ice cream cone fell on the ground and you're just sitting there staring at it and sobbing. As an adult, normally you would know that you can simply go get more ice cream, but after being awake for two days, the mere sight of ice cream on the ground has reduced you to sobbing.
- **At seventy-two hours**, all your higher mental processes are kaput. Concentration, motivation, perception—all useless. Forget coping with dropped ice cream; you can't even get through a basic conversation.

Sometimes, the effects of sleep deprivation can be quite comical, like when I recently spread antibiotic ointment instead of toothpaste on my toothbrush. Fortunately, I'm able to have a good laugh in those moments. I may take my job seriously, but I don't take myself too seriously.

Funny as my antibiotic ointment toothpaste incident may be, here's the bottom line on sleep deprivation. For every twenty-four hours of sleep deprivation, your body's performance declines by 25 percent.[21] Imagine living your life like that, each day running at only 75 percent the capacity you were the previous day. Eventually, you wouldn't be very good for anything!

---

21   J. R. Thorpe, "What Happens to Your Body When You Don't Sleep," *Bustle*, February 12, 2016,
     https://www.bustle.com/articles/140910-what-happens-to-your-body-when-you-dont-sleep.

FINAL SLEEP THOUGHTS

There you have it: everything about sleep that I could fit into one chapter. Before I let you go, I want to give you one final note on sleep deprivation.

In Mary's story, I recommended that she get off sleeping pills to pursue more natural means of healthful sleep. But just to be clear, I'm not opposed to doctor-prescribed medication where necessary—quite the opposite, in fact. It is simply that I encourage you to use the lowest effective dose possible and for the shortest duration. Allowing your body to fall asleep without sedating drugs that change your sleep depth is the ideal way to get restorative rest.

Building healthy habits around the four pillars in this book is a natural, effective way of improving your overall well-being. However, if you don't feel like things are working the way they're supposed to, especially if you start experiencing signs of severe depression or anxiety, seek help right away.[22]

Similarly, in your life, there may be times when you need to go on medication, either temporarily or permanently, and that's okay. The most important thing is that you understand the severity of any health issues you are expe-

---

22 Snoring note: If you or your partner snore loudly and have periods of time when you pause while breathing, these are signs of sleep apnea, a health condition that can have dangerous and deadly consequences. See your doctor right away so you can undergo sleep testing.

riencing. Take medication if you need it, and remember that healthy lifestyle changes can help those medications do their job. They don't have to be mutually exclusive! Eventually, you may be able to improve your underlying physiology to the point where you may be able to change, reduce, or eliminate some of your medications—but only after discussing everything with your doctor, of course.

MARY COMMITS TO BETTER SLEEP

Mary is starting to figure out her passion and goals. Her whole life, she's always done a million things for everybody else. When the kids went to bed, she was up late doing laundry and watching TV. She never developed good sleep habits. She never realized the importance of sleep. Even normal days saw several cups of coffee, and bad days were supplemented with a quad shot at Starbucks.

Mary once read somewhere that as people age, they need less sleep, which isn't true. In fact, impaired function and minor signs of dementia in elderly people are often linked to poor sleep. However, because of this false information, she doesn't worry about the late nights, though she is worried at how much she's come to rely on sleeping pills to help her doze off.

Despite the sleep problems, Mary has started improving

her eating and exercising habits, though she's surprised to discover she's not getting the expected results. She swears she read somewhere that exercise boosts energy, but that hasn't been the case for her at all.

Eventually, she reads another article about all the different ways sleep affects the body, and suddenly a light goes off. The diet and exercise are great healthy habits, but she's been inadvertently holding herself back. She decides it's time to trade in the sleeping pills for more natural remedies, particularly good sleep hygiene.

Because Mary has embraced the SMARTER Goals system and is focused on becoming a healthier person, first she sits down and objectively looks at her usual routine. Quickly she realizes she's only getting five or six hours a night. She rises at about seven every day, but then she's up until one or two every night in front of the TV, on the phone, or on Facebook connecting with her kids. To top it off, her room is warm and filled with bright lights. Now that she understands a little more, she commits to changing her routine.

MARY'S TOP TEN HEALTHY SLEEP TIPS

To make sure she's sound asleep instead of posting funny cat videos at one in the morning, Mary has come up with the following sleep hygiene strategies for her Habit That lifestyle. Feel free to borrow any of these for your own five-minute health-ups!

#1. NO ELECTRONICS IN THE BEDROOM

People are getting about an hour less sleep than they did even two decades ago. In this way, Mary has been part of a larger cultural phenomenon. In the past, when it got dark, people went to sleep because they had nothing else to do. In the electric era, everything changed, and people began ignoring their circadian rhythms.

The blue lights on the LED screens found on smartphones, TVs, and computer screens have only accelerated this process. Our brains perceive blue light as a form of daylight, which tells us it's time to be awake—thus overriding, interfering with, and confusing natural body signals. We might be tired, and our brains know we've been up for a while, but if we perceive daylight, none of that matters.

Mary learns that she should be cutting off screen time a full two hours before bed. But considering the habits she's trying to rewire, that doesn't feel realistic. She still allows herself plenty of screen time, but she's also built herself a bigger buffer by creating a better pre-sleep routine. Sometimes, a text can interrupt her routine and she'll check her phone, but she's starting to use the "do not disturb" function more and more often.

#2. COOL THE ROOM

Mary used to keep the heat on all night because she wanted to be comfortable. Now, she shuts the heat off in the evening and lets her room get down to the low sixties. If that means throwing open a window—yes, even if it's snowing outside—she does it.

These days, Mary has learned all about melatonin, and she knows that if she's going to benefit from this internally produced wonder drug, she has to make the room cool, dark, and quiet.

She thought it would be tough cooling the room down like this, but she's found that it actually makes her bed more appealing since she gets to hunker down under her fluffy blankets.

#3. HAVE A HOT SHOWER OR BATH BEFORE BED

To start the cooling-off process, Mary takes a hot shower before bed. She used to shower in the morning to help wake her up, but since she's less groggy to start her day now, she doesn't mind the trade-off. Just a cool splash of water on her face in the morning, and she's ready to face her day!

#4. TURN OUT THE LIGHTS

The phone and TV are gone from Mary's room. She's even started turning her clock away, accepting that she doesn't need to know what time it is until her alarm goes off. Mary admits that getting rid of the electronics was tough, but she rewarded herself with a new set of curtains that not only look good, but also help make the room darker.

#5. CREATE QUIET OR GET A WHITE NOISE MACHINE

Cool, dark, and quiet doesn't need to be complete silence. Mary's found that if it's too quiet, every little sound outside or in the house ends up distracting her. So, she got a fan for her bedroom and a white noise machine for when she travels.

Mary used to find sleep even more elusive when she was out of town visiting friends and family. Everything sounded different, and it would take her as much as three days to get comfortable. The white noise machine helps that—plus, the sounds of rain on the ocean let her focus her thoughts and drift off to sleep.

#6. HAVE A BEDTIME RITUAL

Bedtime rituals don't have to be complex. Mary previously didn't have any routine whatsoever, save for making her kids' lunches at night. She used to just brush her teeth and lounge around until she zonked out. Now, she does some light stretching, takes a warm shower, brushes her teeth, and then sits to read a book for a little bit. Overall, she's found her new routine naturally helps remove distractions (like those pesky blue-light electronics) and gradually prepares her body for bed.

#7. USE THE SAME SCENT TO REMIND YOURSELF OF BEDTIME

Mary always liked scented candles, but she never thought they'd be helpful for getting to sleep. Now, when she sits down to read, Mary lights her favorite candle to create a pleasant, relaxing environment. She looks forward to this moment each night, and she's come to associate the scent with sleep.

#8. SET AN ALARM FOR BEDTIME

Historically, starting her bedtime routine—or even deciding to go to bed—had been the biggest problem for Mary. She always had one more thing to do in the evening—surfing the web, watching TV, scrapbooking, you name it. Now she's committed to a routine, and her bedtime alarm cues her to get started and allow herself a full eight-hour sleep opportunity.

#9. GIVE YOURSELF A GOOD SLEEP AFFIRMATION

Mary is a healthy person. She's been giving herself that positive affirmation every day for weeks—and she's totally owning the idea.[23]

In the process, she came to realize all the negative affirmations she's told herself about sleep. She'd always told everyone she was a terrible sleeper and that she didn't know how she managed to get out of bed every day. Not anymore.

As soon as that bedtime alarm goes off and Mary begins her routine, she starts telling herself, "I'm a good sleeper. I get restful sleep. I'm ready for my body to relax." Not only does it make her feel better, but it's been effective in helping her mind wind down, too.

#10. KEEP A NOTEBOOK BY THE BED FOR IDEAS

Even with all these great new sleep hygiene strategies, some nights Mary just can't turn her brain off. Her thoughts often feel like a roomful of crazed toddlers sugared up after a birthday party. She used to try shoving those wired toddler thoughts into a closet, but they were

---

23 Just like the idea of affirmations to set your intention for sleep, check out *The Miracle Morning*, by Hal Elrod. His book extolls the virtues of getting up early and having a routine. You will be better at mastering this if you get enough sleep. Check out this amazing book and his online community on Facebook to meet like-minded morning people.

noisy in there, too, plus they kept rearranging things. Now, she lets them all out, accepts them, and gives each a hug.

To do this, Mary allows herself to turn on a dim, yellow light, grab the notebook by her bed, and get all her thoughts out of her brain. That way, she knows all those errant thoughts are in a safe place and she won't forget them. As she turns the light back off, she quietly says, "Thank you, brain, for letting me know. I've got it all on the list. Now it's time for bed."

CHAPTER 6

BURN

I had finished my normal workout at the gym, but the clock said I had ten more minutes before I needed to leave to pick up my kids. Since I had a few minutes to kill and didn't feel completely fatigued, I figured I'd get on the squat press machine and do some light reps at seventy pounds.

My back felt a little sore after a few reps, but I didn't think anything of it. When I stepped out from the machine, though, I realized I could barely walk. In just a few presses at a light weight, I had somehow slipped a disc in my back. Ouch!

Okay, I thought to myself, *this can't be too bad. It will go away in a few days.* I'd never slipped a disc before, though I had broken some bones—my hand, my arm, a couple of ribs, and my tailbone (though thankfully not all at once). At worst, I figured I'd be back to my normal routine in one or two weeks.

Soon, I could see quite clearly how wrong I had been. The next day, I hobbled into a staff meeting and gave a stiff, awkward, and rigid presentation, trying not to move at all. I couldn't lift my kids. I could barely walk, let alone work out. I was miserable. Having medical knowledge isn't reassuring in cases like this; as bad as this was, I knew the course of healing could take six weeks or longer. "Six weeks of *this*?" I wailed. "Ain't nobody got time for that!"

Like most muffin moments (remember that meme from earlier?), the timing was bad. This injury interfered with everything in my life. I was taking care of my mother-in-law with pancreatic cancer, relishing active time with my kids, and becoming more involved at work. Nothing I tried helped. Bed rest made it worse, and too much exercise made it worse, too.[24] I began feeling like a failure. I could see why others in similar situations could lose faith in achieving their own goals.

---

24 Want to know a funny thing about back pain? As it turns out, bed rest can actually make it worse by causing your supporting muscles to weaken. When that happens, the pain gets worse, too. On the other hand, overexercising can stress tissue and delay healing. If you ever slip your disc or otherwise injure your back, your job will be to find that happy balance. Speaking of, if you're not sure if your back injury requires medical attention, here are some signs that you should probably go to the ER: numbness, (especially in the groin), weakness, difficulty urinating, inability to control your bowels and bladder, and inability to walk. Also, falls from heights and severe enough force to break bones should be evaluated, too!

Finally, I accepted that a big old muffin had come between me and my healthy habits. It was frustrating and painful, but I had to look at the big picture. I was a healthy person, and I had to take care of myself. Instead of resisting my new reality, I changed my goals to match my new needs, although there were some curse words along the way—I'm not perfect!

First and foremost, that meant a lot of physical therapy. At first, I only had enough of a pain window for about five minutes of work, but I kept reminding myself if that was all I could manage, I was still meeting my goal and allowing the rehabilitation process to run its course.

I had to start from scratch, building back all the muscle I'd lost in what felt like a never-ending process. If my goal had just been about my body size, or just been about exercising, the temptation to quit would have been too great. However, because my goal was to be a healthy person, I knew that if I was still moving forward, I wasn't a failure.

EXERCISE SHOULDN'T BE INTIMIDATING

There's an old expression, "If there's something that you want to do, you'll find a way; if you don't want to do it, you'll find an excuse." I thought of this saying a lot as I recovered from my slipped disc, and I quote it every time someone mentions their fear of exercise.

I get why people feel intimidated by gyms. I once saw a gym rat stop to kiss his biceps after every set of curls—which was not only an incredible display of narcissism, but also a great way of making us mere mortals feel like we don't belong. Guys like that only confirm our worst fears of the gym in particular, and exercise in general. When we think of the gym, we picture a bunch of hard-body models effortlessly lifting massive barbells and admiring themselves in the mirror.

While some ridiculous people actually do this, that's not how it works at most gyms. My gym, for instance, is filled with a bunch of super-old guys who are just trying to stay healthy. If you walk into your typical gym, you'll likely see the same thing: regular people of all shapes, ages, and sizes.

Most gyms make specific efforts to not be intimidating places, but the truth is you don't need a gym to be a healthy person. We're conditioned to think we need all this fancy workout equipment to exercise properly. We pay for gym memberships we don't use or buy fancy home exercise equipment that sits around collecting dust and stray laundry. Our intentions are good, but we're never going to use these things if they make us feel afraid.

In this chapter, I want to take exercise down a peg or two to make it accessible to you and who you are right now.

When it comes to exercise, just about anything works as long as you're moving. It could be a home Bowflex, it could be a gym membership, or it could be a pair of running shoes. It could be a polished set of videos or some grainy YouTube tutorials from someone that you can relate to. It could even just be a walk around the block or a commitment to take the stairs rather than the elevator. As long as you're doing something, even if it's only five minutes a day, your body will see the benefit. Remember, five minutes of something is better than twenty-four hours of nothing!

WHY EXERCISE IS SO GREAT

What if I could give you a pill that made your brain and organs function better; that improved mood and coordination; that reduced risk of chronic pain, fibromyalgia, depression, anxiety, heart disease, ADD, and ADHD; that made you look better; and that improved muscle tone and libido? What if I promised there were no adverse side effects either?

Okay, you got me. Just like in the last chapter, there's no magic pill for any of this (which is sad—I was really hoping for that pet unicorn and tropical island home!). However, exercise is a pretty magical drug.

Our bodies are designed to move. When we don't grant

our bodies this simple request, a lot of pesky problems start to creep in. It's true that the last thing anyone wants to do when they feel bad is exercise, yet it's the very thing that will get you on the path to feeling better.

The great thing is you don't need a lot of exercise to start feeling the benefits. All you have to do is start moving. The question is, what's the best way to get going?

NERD ALERT: HEALTHY EXERCISES

With all this talk about exercise, you're probably thinking to yourself, "This is all great, but when is Dr. Hope actually going to tell me which exercises to do?" First off, according to the Habit That lifestyle, any exercise that can be performed safely that you will actually stick to is a good exercise to do. If all you have is five minutes in your day to practice a few lunges or run up and down some stairs, then that's an excellent exercise to be doing during that time. Five minutes is better than no minutes!

However, the best exercises are the ones that you enjoy and that fit in with your SMARTER Goals. When seeking out the right workouts for yourself, here are some things to consider.

High-Intensity Interval Training (HIIT)
Increasing clinical studies are demonstrating that HIIT can

be an effective alternative to long endurance-type training.[25] This is great news for those of us mere mortals who don't run Ironman triathlons before breakfast each day! In fact, a study in *Exercise and Sport Science Reviews* showed that six weeks of HIIT can improve metabolism and endurance.[26]

How do you do it? Well, the amounts of time vary depending on which exercise you follow, but the basic idea is to alternate between a limited time of all-out, incredibly intense exercise (sprinting, burpees, jumps, etc.) and very brief periods of rest. Because this bust/rest cycle doesn't let your body fully recover, you can achieve greater metabolic gains.[27]

The Tabata workout is a good example. In this exercise, participants move between twenty seconds of intense exercise and ten seconds of rest for a cycle of two minutes. After a more generous recovery period, you can choose to perform additional cycles. In one workout, the twenty-second exercises could include jumping lunges, burpees, high knees, and mountain climbers. You can also download apps with timers and create your own!

25 Martin J. Gibala, Jonathan P. Little, Maureen J. MacDonald, and John A. Hawley, "Physiological Adaptations to Low-Volume, High-Intensity Interval Training in Health and Disease," *The Journal of Physiology*, January 30, 2012, https://doi.org/10.1113/jphysiol.2011.224725.

26 Martin J. Gibala and Sean L. McGee, "Metabolic Adaptations to Short-term High-Intensity Interval Training: A Little Pain for a Lot of Gain?" *Exercise and Sport Science Reviews* 2, no. 36 (2008): 58–63, doi:10.1097/JES.0b013e318168ec1f.

27 Paul B. Laursen and David G. Jenkins, "The Scientific Basis for High-Intensity Interval Training," *Sports Medicine* 32, no. 1 (November 2, 2012): 53–73, https://link.springer.com/article/10.2165/00007256-200232010-00003.

Tabata training, named after Japanese scientist Dr. Izumi Tabata from the National Institute of Fitness and Sports in Tokyo, is a studied form of HIIT.[28] The research team divided athletes into two groups. Group one trained with moderate intensity for one hour, five days per week. Group two trained with HIIT exercises for four minutes and twenty seconds, four days per week. That's five hours per week versus seventeen minutes! After six weeks, both groups saw improvements (of course!), but group two enjoyed more significant gains! The key here is the intensity. Interval training has to be very intense in order to reap the benefits. Half-assed jumping jacks won't cut it.

Cardiovascular Exercise

Cardiovascular exercise—often referred to as "cardio" or the more old-school "aerobics"—includes running, jumping jacks, swimming, burpees (yep, they're great for both HIIT and cardio!), mountain climbers, vigorous dancing, cycling, and using gym machines, such as treadmills, stair climbers, and elliptical machines. If you're looking for a way to gauge your necessary level of difficulty, cardio exercise should leave you feeling short of breath and having difficulty carrying on a conversation. However, if you are experiencing chest pain or are too short of breath to function, you are overdoing it!

While great for burning calories, cardio has other benefits

---

28   Talisa Emberts, John Porcari, Scott Dobers-tein, Jeff Steffen, and Carl Foster, "Exercise Intensity and Energy Expenditure of a Tabata Workout," *Journal of Sports Science and Medicine* 12, no. 3 (2013): 612–613, https://www.ncbi.nlm.nih.gov/pmc/articles/PMC3772611/.

as well, such as improved lung and heart strength, increased circulation, elimination of excess stress hormones, elevated mood, decreased depression, improved energy, and maybe even decreased risk of cancer.[29]

How do you find the right cardio exercise for you? For this one, the best answer is a question. Which one sounds like fun? If you love dancing, put on a fast song and get moving! If you're more of a swimming, biking, or hiking person, that's great, too. Do whatever you'll actually want to do. After all, it doesn't matter how great an exercise is if you hate it and never actually go through with it.

For instance, I could tell you all day about how great burpees are as a calorie scorcher. But I won't burn many calories telling you about it—nor will you burn many just by listening to me. To do it right, you gotta get up (and down).[30] Again, five minutes (or more) of any exercise you like is better than zero minutes of an exercise you hate. Try a few, mix it up, add a soundtrack or some friends, and start getting your heart rate up!

---

29 There is substantial medical evidence that cardio reduces the risk of several cancers, including colon cancer, breast cancer, and uterine cancer. This is thought to be due to how exercise reduces weight and inflammation, as well as improving immune function. For more information on the exercise-cancer reduction connection, check out https://www.cancer.gov/about-cancer/causes-prevention/risk/obesity/physical-activity-fact-sheet.

30 If you're not familiar with burpees, here are the basics. Invented by Royal H. Burpee (yes, that was a real person), burpees are a full-body exercise that have you begin in a standing position, move into a squat with your hands on the ground, kick your feet back into plank position (where you can add a push-up if you're feeling extra vigorous that day), return your feet back to squat position, and then jump up to standing. Check out a video on YouTube to see how to do this great free exercise! To learn more about its history, check out this *Huffington Post* article: https://www.huffingtonpost.com/2014/05/02/burpee-history_n_5248575.html.

Weight Training

All right, ladies, don't skip this section! Lifting a few dumb-bells isn't going to turn you into a big, beefy body builder! Strengthening muscle makes you look leaner and tightens areas of your body. You don't have to be an Olympic strong-man to get the benefits, and you won't bulk up like the people you see on TV without insanely intense training and some other "enhancements," so don't fear the free-weight section of the gym!

Lifting a weight stresses your muscles and bones. In this case, though, it is good stress! The activity causes increased blood flow to the areas getting action, increasing the nutri-ent supply and enhancing performance. As your muscles get stronger, your stamina improves. Meanwhile, your bones are also getting stronger, which decreases your risk of fractures.

Best of all, you don't have to lift anchors or giant tires to get the benefits. You can do bodyweight exercises such as squats and push-ups—or you can just lift things around the house, such as gallon jugs of water or your kids.

It doesn't have to be either/or. You can combine strength training with cardio. Do some burpees and kettlebell swings, and you will see how well these strength builders get your heart rate up and your lungs working. You can take many strength-based exercises and speed them up to get the cardio boost. Or, if you are using dumbbells for your arms, walk around or go on the treadmill to boost the benefits. Just be mindful of form and safety; you don't want to pull a muscle or fall! Your goal is to be a healthy person, not a patient in my ER!

Whatever form of exercise you choose, you will start to see benefits. You will feel more confident, your mood will improve, and you'll look and feel great—all while fighting off dementia and other chronic illnesses! Even if you only have five minutes on a busy day, getting your body moving will get you closer to your goals.

HERE'S HOW TO HABIT THAT

If you're considering starting or ramping up an exercise routine, first, know that it's almost always safe and healthy to exercise. People with spotty medical history often worry about this. They'll say, "I've had a heart attack before, so I don't know if exercise is safe. Won't it cause another heart attack?" In fact, the opposite is true. The only way to decrease your risk of a future heart attack is to get healthier—and you get healthier through exercise.

As we've said throughout this book, though, you start where you start. If your arteries are 99 percent clogged and you're at risk of another heart attack, I'm not going to suggest you hop on a treadmill. If you are in that situation, you can get started with cardiac rehab supervised by a medical professional, which would allow you to slowly increase your muscle strength and move on to more demanding activities. Here are some other things to keep in mind as you get started.

FIND YOUR BASELINE

For babies, their baseline is zero. They can't walk, they can't talk, they can't feed themselves, they can't do anything. They don't start as Olympic athletes, but as they ramp up into functioning people, they could become Olympians eventually.

Naturally, you're not a baby (and if you are, congratulations on learning how to read at such a young age!). The point, however, is that you understand where your health currently is and what your limitations are. I hurt my back and couldn't perform my usual routine of vigorous exercise or lifting. Our friend George has a bad knee and can't run. Luckily, running isn't his goal; becoming a healthier person is. Where you start is where you start— and sometimes muffins will happen and require you to start all over.

DON'T OVERDO IT

"Squatting two-hundred pounds while standing on a yoga ball: this is why emergency rooms exist."

Whatever you can do in your current context, start with that and slowly increase toward your goal. If you try to push beyond that, you could end up injuring yourself and throwing yourself off track.

I've had patients who overdid it. Some patients experienced such extreme muscle protein breakdown that it clogged up their blood and kidneys and forced them into the hospital, where they were put on IV fluids in an attempt to stave off permanent kidney damage and the need for dialysis. Other patients I've seen hadn't exercised in years, but they suddenly decided to become mega ultra-power lifters, throwing out their backs, breaking their legs, or pulling hamstrings in the process. You don't go from zero to Greek god overnight!

Even accomplished athletes have to watch out on this one. I have nothing against people who participate in marathons or Ironmans, but sometimes their hardcore and body-punishing attitudes aren't healthy. There's a saying in these communities that, "You're not really a marathon runner until you've had bloody diarrhea." That's not the attitude of a healthy person.

Since crapping blood is usually something to be avoided, I encourage you to find that big, broad sweet spot between bloody stool and sitting on a couch eating doughnuts. Put a little more politely, your exercises should be grounded but ambitious. After you exercise, you should feel a bit winded, a bit of a work on your muscles, and a bit of an ache in your body. You don't want to suffer, but some stress is good; it's how your body grows. That means walking from the couch to the refrigerator probably isn't going to cut it.

In the eighties, pushing yourself outside of your comfort zone was often referred to as "feeling the burn." Every time I start a jog, I can feel that burn kick in once I get to the end of my quarter-mile road. That's when the change in my breathing happens. It's easy to want to quit at this starting point, but that's your body doing the work it's supposed to. If you can push past that, you can get in the groove. That's where the real fun (and benefit!) starts.

Again, a word of caution here. You're supposed to be feeling something; however, if your body hurts, or if you're experiencing extreme stress or chest pain, then stop and talk to your doctor. And another word of caution: be careful when you try something new—and don't forget to exercise your common sense!

NERD ALERT: WHEN TO SEE A DOCTOR

When should you see a doctor, and what kind of doctor should you see? My patients often have a lot of uncertainty around these questions, so let's take a moment to address some basic concerns.

Visit your primary care doctor for:

- Colds
- Yearly checkups
- Checking your cholesterol
- Mild discomfort that's not interfering with your life, but you have questions
- Screening exams
- Colonoscopies
- Getting clearance to start an exercise program

Visit an emergency room if you have:

- Chest pains (especially made worse with exercise)
- Trouble breathing
- Signs of an allergic reaction
- Bleeding that won't stop (from any part of your body)
- Broken bones or dislocated joints
- Signs of a stroke (facial drooping, difficulty with speech, difficulty using one side of your body)
- Fainting or loss of consciousness
- Sudden changes in vision or loss of vision
- Confusion or change in level of consciousness
- Severe or persistent vomiting
- Coughing or vomiting up blood
- Uncontrolled infections
- Any severe trauma or head injury
- Suicidal or homicidal feelings

Some of these may sound obvious to you. However, I've seen firsthand that it's not. Some patients come to the ER for every fresh cold that hits them (and we aren't withholding the miracle cure for colds...there isn't one!). Others will break an arm and calmly wait a week to meet with their primary care doctor. My general advice is this: if you're wondering whether you should see a doctor, you probably should. We never turn anyone away. It's better to be evaluated for something minor than to let something major go unchecked—especially in cases where time is of the essence.

MAKE IT WORK FOR YOU

Get bored during workouts and want to quit? Try using different methods to distract yourself from the hard work of it:

- If you're jogging, plan your loop in advance or create alternate routes.
- Let yourself daydream.
- Listen to music, podcasts, or an audiobook.
- Watch TV while you are on a treadmill.

There are plenty of ways to make it work for you, even if that means finding activities that are so fun they don't feel like working out, such as dancing. Anything you enjoy that moves your muscles and leaves you somewhat winded counts. This is especially good to know if you're not ready for a vigorous exercise program quite yet. If that's the case, just remember that even things like mowing the lawn, gardening, and cleaning the house can count as activity, since they get you moving and require sustained effort.

My four-year-old and six-year-old have found plenty of active shenanigans. In fact, they love deciding what's exercise and what isn't. So far, they've determined that jumping up and down and whacking the couch with a sword are both exercise, but that sleeping isn't. Also, riding bikes is, but swinging really isn't. I'm always happy to participate in these activities with them, too. Nothing wrong with making exercise fun!

In fact, exercising with other people has additional benefits, whether you're leaping with your kids, going for a walk with a friend, participating in team sports, meeting somebody at the gym, doing a group fitness class, or joining a dance class at your local community center. You'll always get a nice dose of feel-good endorphins from exercise, but when you've got partners, you'll get an even greater social-connection oxytocin rush than you would if you exercised by yourself.

Plus, social exercise creates greater accountability and helps you push yourself harder. I may think I'm pushing it when I'm by myself, but I've found the collective energy in my workout classes always takes me to the next level. The leader in one of my classes is such a nonstop, happy, high-energy type that I can't help but feel great on the way out, no matter how hard he just pushed me. Plus he sings and tells goofy jokes to keep the mood light and fun.

NERD ALERT: EXERCISE INCREASES METABOLISM?

Metabolism is the biochemical process through which your body turns food into energy. This involves breathing, digestion, delivering nutrients to your cells via your bloodstream, use of energy by your cells (nerves transmitting signals, muscles contracting, etc.), and elimination of the by-products of metabolism (waste).

These biochemical reactions occur via the reduction-oxidation reactions of the tricarboxylic acid cycle (also known as the Krebs cycle), which is how the body makes ATP (adenosine triphosphate), which you can think of as the currency of the body. Cells use ATP like money to get what they want. Some processes are more expensive than others (such as exercise) and burn more ATP money. Less expensive processes, like sleeping, use less ATP.

At any rate, your body is never *not* burning calories. Yup, even during your most chill Netflix binge, you are burning calories just breathing, circulating blood, and surviving—but not much, so don't start counting binge-watching as exercise (especially if triple-cheese pizza is involved). Your basal metabolic rate is what you need for your basic essential functions.

When most people talk about metabolism, they usually aren't nerding out about adenosine triphosphate like we are here. They are usually referring to the rate at which your body burns calories. Thin people often thank their "good" metabolism, while overweight people often blame their "bad" metabolism. But the awesome thing is that you have the power to improve your metabolism! Here are a few biochemical truths you can use!

1. Muscle burns more calories than fat. Just to live and function, a muscle cell burns more calories than a fat cell. How much more is up for debate. But the bottom line is this: the more you use your muscles, the more your metabolism increases.

2. High-intensity interval training burns extra calories long after the workout is over. Combining intensity and strength will increase the benefits even further![31]

3. Skipping meals can actually *lower* your metabolism. Imagine that you are a camel. You are going through the desert,

31 Paige Waehner, "Make Small Changes for Big Results," *VeryWellFit*, February 18, 2018, https://www.verywellfit.com/secret-weapons-of-weight-loss-1231575.

where water is scarce. So you store up excess fluid in your available space—mostly your humps—because your body has learned to hold on to every drop. Now imagine you skip meals for most of the day (sending your body the message that food is scarce), and then have a large, heavy meal that evening. Your body will store the excess calories in your available space, fat cells, because your body has learned to hold on to every calorie. Remember, it is your metabolism's job to keep you alive, not to care about how your abs look!

SOME PRACTICAL APPROACHES TO EXERCISE

If you've become inactive, it can be difficult to make exercise a part of your life. If that's the case, you might try incorporating multiple things together, instead of trying to fit everything into a busy schedule. For instance, it's a lot easier to find time to exercise and be with your kids if you combine both into one activity. Or, if you work a lot, it's a lot easier to get yourself moving if you make it part of your routine. Here are some pointers to get you going.

INCORPORATE EXERCISE INTO YOUR LIFE

I attended a Genius Network Annual Event Conference where one of the featured speakers, billionaire Naveen Jain, talked about how he would sometimes bring his kids to meetings so they could see how he negotiated. As a result, they learned how to treat people with respect, even during intense emotional moments.[32]

I sat in the audience and thought, *I'm not negotiating multimillion-dollar deals, but I bet I can incorporate my kids into parts of my life that can help teach them valuable lessons.* (They frown on bringing children in to watch the gore of the trauma bay in the emergency department, so exercising with them *outside* of work seems like a better plan than Bring Your Kid to Work Day.) I had exercised with them before, but not consistently. Usually, I would only work out while they were napping or at school, but with other to-dos like household chores, grocery shopping, work, and writing this book, I began to wonder if I could fit exercise into a different part of my day. After listening to Naveen Jain, I realized that exercise was a great way to spend quality time with my kids and serve as a positive role model for them at the same time. I've been able to teach them that exercise is fun and that our family values health and strength, while reinforcing my own goals.

Remember, young kids especially have limitless energy. The more you encourage them, the more they'll see

---

32 In case you're curious about Naveen Jain, here's the short version: he's a self-made billionaire dude who cofounded InfoSpace (now Blucora, an internet services company) back in the day and now helps run a space program called Moon Express. He's also a pretty fun speaker if you ever get the chance to watch him.

exercise as an appropriate way to burn that energy. Plus, they'll make it look so fun that you'll want to join in.

For instance, one day after my son finished both school and then an hour-long gymnastics class, he still had more energy than he knew what to do with. As we stood in the lobby waiting for his sister to finish *her* gymnastics class, I used his energy as an opportunity.

"Quick!" I told him. "Hop on your left foot fifteen times! Now do ten jumping jacks! Run around like a lion!"

Our activity attracted all the other kids who were also waiting for their siblings, and soon about seven other kids were following my commands. As a result, I got to exercise with my kid and a bunch of random little strangers just because I saw an opportunity to keep my child engaged. It was a time-effective exercise, and a great way of incorporating activity into my life—although now these same kids expect new entertaining exercises and activities every week. I've created little health monsters!

BURN TO FOCUS

In the United States, we expect children to sit still and learn all day long. But schools in some other countries get their children up and running every forty-five minutes. In one article I read about this, one educator was asked how they could get any teaching done in such an environment. The way the educator saw it, however, frequent activity was the *only* way to actually get any teaching done.[33]

What works for school works for work, too. As adults, we often sit at our desks all day. However, there's a limit to how much you can concentrate, even with a good night's sleep (which you're now getting thanks to those SMARTER Goals you set, right?). To be more productive at work, get your body moving. Walk up and down the stairs a few times, do ten burpees or jumping jacks, or take a walk around the block to get some fresh air. Physical activity helps increase the blood flow to all parts of your body, including your brain, and it can also help stimulate your energy and reset your perspective.

People often worry about taking even five- or ten-minute breaks. However, just like when you commit to sleeping instead of pulling all-nighters, these little breaks are shown to be incredibly beneficial. Remember, the Habit That life is built around these little five-minute opportunities for quick wins. Set an alarm every two hours to allow yourself to get up and move. You'll feel better, you'll be more productive, and you'll reinforce your healthy habits by incorporating them into your day.

---

33 For more on these programs, see Patrick Butler, "No grammar schools, lots of play: The secrets of Europe's top education system," *The Guardian*, September 20, 2016, https://www.theguardian.com/education/2016/sep/20/grammar-schools-play-europe-top-education-system-finland-daycare.

DON'T GO OUT OF YOUR WAY

If every day requires a monumental effort to get your workout in, then you're probably not going to stick to your intended routine very long. For instance, are you really going to go to a gym that's an hour's drive away? Are you really going to wake up at 5:00 a.m. for a jog if you're not a morning person?

Instead of literally going out of your way to exercise, incorporate it into your life as it is right now. The more you bring exercise into your comfort zone, the easier it will be to make it consistent and habitual.

This also applies to the frequency of exercise. If you haven't exercised in five years, then trying to work out five days a week might be asking a little much. Find something that's realistic for you when you're making your SMARTER Goals.

MAKE IT ROUTINE

As I've said throughout the book, the more choices you can remove from your cognitive load, the more likely you are to stick with them. If you have to think about your exercise and make a separate decision each time, then each time you're giving yourself the opportunity to say no. Routines set you free.

My dad is one of the calmest, steadiest, and most consistent people I have ever met. He goes to the gym at least three times per week without fail. Whenever we joke that he'd still show up even if the gym burned down, he agrees.

Not too long ago, he had a chance to prove his commitment to routine. His gym didn't burn down, but it did change owners, and he didn't like the way they ran things. Without missing a beat, he simply started going to a different gym. Quitting never occurred to him. His goal was to be a healthy person, not work out at a specific gym. The minor course correction couldn't derail this committed guy! Triceps day will not be stopped!

LET THE LITTLE THINGS ADD UP

Five minutes of something is better than zero minutes of nothing. One-hour blocks of exercise are great, but they're not the only option for effective exercise. Each activity builds up over time. Maybe you can't exercise after work, but you can find time for jumping jacks or jogs up and down the stairs.

Naturally, you know your life better than I do, so you'll be able to come up with better ideas for yourself than I can. The point is, there are so many ways to incorporate movement into your life that you can't go wrong as long as you get started.

START WHERE YOU ARE

When it comes to exercise, people often say things like, "Oh, I'm not as fast, fit, strong, or thin as I used to be." Who cares? This is where you are—not there, but here. It's okay to start here and get there eventually. Whatever you can do at your current level is what I want you to do—though I also want you to make sure you're pushing yourself. Whatever that may be, all I ask is that you own it and love it.

I don't say this to make you feel better; I say it to remove obstacles and objections. If the only time you can exercise is when your favorite TV airs, that's fine. Supplement your TV habit with an exercise habit. It could look something like this:

- Set a timer that goes off every five minutes. For the first five minutes, march in place. For the second five minutes, lunge side-to-side and then front and back.
- During commercial breaks, do something more vigorous, like jumping jacks or a few laps up and down the stairs.
- Spend the last two minutes of the show with a gentle stretch or movement.

Something is better than nothing. Your workout doesn't have to be an intense aerobics class to be effective. The more you roll exercise in with your TV habit, the more you'll associate them together, helping you to feel empowered and in control of your body. If you want, you can build from there. A lot of modern gyms have TVs on their treadmills, helping you to ramp up your workouts without sacrificing something else you love in the process.

DON'T FOCUS ON EXERCISE GEAR AND GIMMICKS

Don't buy what you don't need. You don't need the latest infomercial gadget, especially if you're just beginning. You can do squats, lunges, jumping jacks, and burpees using only your body weight at home. If you prefer some gear, you'll likely find small hand weights or weighted stretch bands are great starting points.

Don't forget, YouTube is free. They've got everything—cardio, dance, great-butt workouts, ab workouts, jumping-up-and-down-in-crazy-outfits workouts, arm workouts, you name it. Look up trainers or specific subjects on YouTube, find some videos that resonate with you, and go for it.

I like my gym. It's an accepting environment filled with plenty of old, overweight people, which is how it's supposed to be. Everyone is there to get healthier, not walk around with a clipboard judging people's butts. At the majority of gyms, there's nothing there to embarrass you.

That said, I get it if gyms aren't for you. Maybe you don't

like the equipment, maybe you don't like paying the membership, or maybe it's too far outside of your current routine. That's why I love reminding people they have great free resources available at home. As you start and get more advanced, if you find that you want to start adding some tools, great! Use them as rewards while setting your SMARTER Goals.

Alternatively, maybe you really have one piece of equipment in mind that you'd like to start with. For instance, maybe you really want to get one of those mini trampolines and do some jumping. Do it, and make it part of your new goal. Tell yourself you're going to jump X days a week on your trampoline while watching your favorite show. I used to do this exercise myself (pre-back injury), and I loved it.

WHAT ABOUT VACATIONS?

To exercise or not to exercise while on vacation? That is the question. Do you break your routine for a week, or do you find the hotel gym and keep going?

It's up to you. If you do take the time off, just get back into it as soon as you get back into your regular environment. I tend to exercise regularly on my trips, mostly because we eat and drink more while on vacation, and those exercises help balance me out (plus, the more I burn, the more I get to eat).

Either way, make the decision ahead of time, and own it. If you decide no, you won't feel guilty about it because you've given yourself permission to skip a week. If you decide yes, it will help you plan how to work it in. Perhaps the vacation spot has fun hiking, snorkeling, or skiing opportunities—then it's not like working out at all!

It's good to consider what you'll do on vacation, just like it's good to consider what you'll do if you become injured. Both are normal stumbling blocks. They happen. Being a healthy person isn't only about exercise. It's about all four pillars. If exercise isn't in the cards for a week, as a healthy person, you still have plenty of other ways to take care of yourself.

WHY EXERCISE IS SO GOOD

Exercise reaps endless benefits. Everything you do is worth it. Even when you're just starting out, your body reacts positively, and the benefits only continue to build from there:

- If you have asthma, exercise improves your lung function within weeks.
- If you have experienced a heart attack or heart problems, and provided your doctor has cleared you for physical activity, exercise will improve your heart function.
- It decreases high blood pressure, decreases the strain

on your blood vessels, and lessens the effects of diabetes.

- If you're a smoker, exercise can help mitigate some of its effects. It also often acts as extra incentive for smokers to cut down or quit.
- Exercise improves your mental function and cognition. Studies show that people who exercise regularly perform better in school and work, display improved coordination and memory, and have decreased incidences of dementia.

Those are all wonderful things, but if we were to simplify it even further, we could say that exercise simply makes us feel better. When joggers say, "You don't understand. I have to run," they aren't entirely exaggerating. After all, the endorphin boost you can get from exercise rivals any drug, providing pain-relieving benefits to your body's natural opioid receptors and reducing your stress hormones.

Remember our discussion of human growth hormone in Chapter 5? While rest helps trigger your HGH burst at night, exercise takes care of you during the day, which actually helps you sleep better in the process (as long as you're not exercising right before bedtime). Exercise also increases testosterone, which serves important functions in both men and women. Oh, and exercise also makes your body look better, which then increases your confidence and helps boost your libido. We all want to look great and be in the mood, and exercise accomplishes that!

NERD ALERT: HOW EXERCISE IMPROVES SEX

Exercise produces a lot of healthy hormones, such as endorphins (nature's morphine) and testosterone, and it also reduces your stress hormone, cortisol (a major bedroom buzzkill). That's already good enough, but it turns out that exercise with a partner has extra benefits.

Exercising with a partner also helps produce the "relationship hormone," oxytocin, which will further boost the feel-good effects and increase your desire. Plus, after a great couple's workout, hitting the shower together is a fun reward for your hard work.

Exercise improves blood flow to all organs, including your genitals. Better circulation leads to better erections, increased engorgement of the clitoris, and a body healthy enough to engage in—and enjoy—sexual activity. The increased blood flow also makes you more sensitive to the touch by bathing your nerve endings in nutrients and oxygen; this increases the effects of sexual stimulation and can lead to better orgasms.

Strength-building exercises increase testosterone, the hormone of arousal in men *and* women. Testosterone is produced in the testicles in men and the ovaries in women. In adults, testosterone helps with production of red blood cells, improves bone density, leads to better fat distribution (away from the gut), improves muscle strength, builds stamina, and improves sex drive. Low testosterone can lead to a myriad of health problems, such as low libido, erectile dysfunction, loss of muscle and bone strength, decreased fertility, fatigue, and decreased energy. Keeping this essential libido-enhancing hormone up with exercise (and adequate sleep, of course) can improve your health along with your love life!

Kegels are a specific exercise where you squeeze the pubo-coccygeus muscles (the ones that help you stop urinating midstream). For women, this is a lifting of the perineum (skin between vagina and anus) and squeezing of the vagina. For men, practice stopping urine midstream and squeeze your pelvic floor up like you are preventing yourself from passing gas. Once you have identified the sensation of the muscle movement, then it's just like any exercise: the more reps you do, the stronger you get!

ALL THAT SUGAR HAS TO GO SOMEWHERE

Just as exercise brings tons of positives, a lack of exercise poses endless dangers to your health. One of the biggest reasons comes down to how your body stores energy.

When you eat things like sugar, it moves around in your

bloodstream like a bunch of teenage hooligans after a soccer match, carelessly knocking into stuff and causing all sorts of damage. Your body then releases insulin to police these sugar hooligans and send them back home so they're not causing any damage.

Catching the sugar is one thing, but then your insulin needs to stow it somewhere. First, the insulin will knock on the door to your muscles and ask, "Is there any room here?"

If you haven't exercised, your muscles will say, "Well, normally we love taking in as many calories as we can get because they make us big and strong. But sadly, we're not really doing much of anything right now, so we've got nowhere to put all that sugar."

The insulin says, "Okay, whatever," and moves on to your fat cells, which always have plenty of room. At the same time, your insulin will also deposit some of that sugar in your liver, which then clogs, loses functionality, and becomes diseased.

NERD ALERT: INJURIES

Ugh. I have definitely been there. My tally of injuries includes broken ribs, a broken left arm, a broken right hand (in two places), a broken tailbone, a concussion, a slipped disc in my lower back, a left knee meniscus tear (got surgery for that one!), various ankle sprains, plenty of contusions, cuts, scrapes, and the occasional bruise to my dignity. Having been on both the patient side and physician side of injuries, here are some important lessons I've learned.

Pay attention to what you are doing! If you are lifting something heavy, be conscious of your form. If you are climbing, be mindful of your footing. If you are walking on ice (that damn slippery cold stuff has been responsible for a number of my injuries, leading me to conclude I should just move to a more tropical locale), go slow and steady. Many injuries occur when we aren't paying complete attention to what we are doing and our bodies' form. Staying focused in the moment when you exercise is a great safety tip and has the added benefit of training your brain in the art and practice of living in the moment.

If you do get injured, don't ignore it! My knee injury got worse and worse because I just *had* to keep going. Of course, I had the typical immortal mindset of a teenager at that time. The older, wiser me (mostly) doesn't do that. Pain is your body's way of telling you something is wrong. Like touching a hot burner, the pain is to get you to stop already, before you make the damage worse. "Feel the burn" doesn't apply here! Your body needs time to heal.

Seek a professional when needed. Fractures, severe cuts, bad sprains, and strains should be evaluated by a doctor. Physical therapy, splinting/casting, and staying off it might be what is best in order to return to optimal function. Remember, your goal is to be a healthy person, not complete one specific task. With a focus on the bigger picture, remind yourself that a temporary setback is merely an inconvenience, just a bump on the road, a muffin moment. Failing to allow proper healing time will lead to being out much longer.

If you injure yourself, get off that part of your body immediately. See if it is deformed (spoiler alert: that is bad) or numb (also bad). Apply ice to reduce swelling and inflammation. For cuts, rinse with water. Do *not* use rubbing alcohol, peroxide, or iodine. These "cures" are myths. They can actually kill the healthy cells you need in order to repair cuts and slow healing. Besides, any one of those things worsens scarring—plus it hurts! Just say no. If bleeding won't stop, apply pressure and proceed to your nearest emergency department.

Return to activity as soon as it is safe. Being off something *too* long can lead to muscle and ligament weakness and make you more prone to reinjury. For ankle sprains, for example, although we don't want you jumping or running on it, you can do gentle exercises to keep it strong and nimble and on the road to recovery. One of my favorite ankle rehab exercises is to use my foot/ankle to draw out the letters of the alphabet. This is great for strengthening to prevent injuries in the sprain-prone too! Gentle return to activity should be guided by a professional and you should stop if the pain gets worse!

FINAL EXERCISE THOUGHTS

Now that you've exercised your brain with some helpful thoughts on exercise, you're almost ready to head off in victory to our final chapter. Before you go, however, I do have one final note: listen to your body and trust what it's saying.

Let me give you an example of what I mean. I was never a runner. I never particularly enjoyed it, and I certainly never understood how anyone could. One day, I said all this to one of my friends, a weirdo runner type who'll pound out six miles just for fun, and he said, "What do you mean you're not a runner? You have two legs. You have the ability to run. Therefore, you are a runner."

I took his bait and started on a "couch to 5K" program. At first, I ran for two minutes and then walked for a minute. Slowly, I ran more and walked less. "Hey, he was right!" I said. "I totally am a runner!"

Some weeks later, though, I started off with tons of energy, ran two miles from my house, and then suddenly my body said, "I am done running right now. I have angered the slipped disc gods and they are about to smite me. I need to respect that and stop." I tried to push it, but it was no use; I had nothing left in the gas tank and my back was screaming for mercy. I came to a stop, let myself catch my breath, and grimaced at the thought of walking the two miles back home. It was anything but convenient, but I reminded myself I was a healthy person, and it was the right thing to do. There is no trophy for hurting yourself!

GEORGE'S TOP TEN EXERCISE TIPS

He wishes it weren't so, but George has realistic limitations in the form of a knee problem. He can't start doing squats or go for a run, but he also knows his knee and other symptoms will feel better if he takes some of the weight off and gets moving.

George is going to prove to his doctor he's a healthy person. Since he can't run or do a ton of weight-bearing exercises, he's found the swimming pool to be a great starting point. That way, he gets some resistance from the water without forcing his knees to bear much of the load. He's tried a little bit of everything in the pool: walking, swimming, and even water-aerobics classes.

Already George is starting to feel some positive benefits, which in turn have made him want to try other things that make sense in his life. It turns out the cumulative effects of small changes really do make a difference! Here are ten activities that George likes to check off his list throughout the day. Which ones will you incorporate into your own health-ups?

#1. TAKE STAIRS INSTEAD OF ELEVATORS

When George started out, he couldn't even walk a mile—and it probably wasn't a great idea, anyway. One day, however, he wondered what if he started taking the stairs wherever he went? It wasn't more than a couple minutes of exercise, but it got him moving and got his heart rate up. To his surprise, it felt good, and he felt energized. "I can do this!" he'd say out loud before climbing another floor. Soon, he began to wonder what other small changes he could make.

#2. PARK FARTHER AWAY

George no longer parks right up front when he's at the supermarket or the hardware store. Instead, he parks farther back in the parking lot and then hoofs it to the entrance. The quick win feels great, affording him another little burst of activity to empower him as he moves forward.

#3. YOU ARE WHAT YOU MEASURE

George isn't really a tech guy, but after his daughter learned about some of his SMARTER Goals, she got him a Fitbit. It was easy to figure out, and George found himself fascinated by the amount of steps he was taking in a day. He even found himself marching in place during *Matlock* just to get his numbers up. Part of him thought the effort was silly, but the uptick in his heart rate confirmed that even marching in place was a step in the right direction.

#4. MAKE IT SOCIAL

George was surprised to learn how much he enjoyed the water aerobics classes. The social environment inspired a feeling of obligation to a larger group—a feeling he's missed since retirement. Plus, the positive pressure helps keep him going. After he missed a week with the flu, his classmates all let him know they missed him and congratulated him for coming back the following week.

Sometimes, just to change things up, George gets a couple of friends together to walk the mall. It keeps him off the icy roads in the winter and helps him with shopping ideas to spoil his grandkids.

#5. MAKE IT A COMPETITION

George's best friend, Hank, is just as stubborn and competitive as George is, and extra cantankerous to boot. When Hank found out about George's fancy new Fitbit, he got jealous and challenged George to a walk-off. Now they have a standing bet to see who can get the most steps in by the end of the month—with the loser buying the winner's dinner.

#6. EXERCISE DOESN'T HAVE TO BE DRUDGERY

George has already tried plenty of exercises that don't work for him. He even went to his daughter's hip-hop dance class one time, though he spent so much time trying to remember the moves and grumbling about the music that he didn't have much fun with it.

Oh well, he thought to himself. *Some things are a fit, and some things are not.* George's tenacity eventually got him into the pool, which he has taken to like a fish to water. To get even with his daughter, he invited her out to one of his water aerobics classes one time, and laughed all the way home as she complained nonstop about the aquatic experience.

#7. SCHEDULE IT LIKE A MEETING AND HAVE YOUR CLOTHES READY

When George first started moving around more, he made a simple calendar that he pinned to the refrigerator. While his retirement left him with plenty of free time, he found that if he didn't plan ahead, he'd forget his goals and fail to make time for them. Once he found the water aerobics, he eagerly penciled the times in each week. For other days, he'd look for blocks of time to take a couple laps around the block and get his step count up to make sure he beat Hank's numbers for the month.

#8. GET A REAL-LIFE TRAINER OR GET A FREE TRAINER ON YOUTUBE

George's daughter suggested he try some YouTube videos for a few exercise tips. Although tech isn't his favorite thing, he managed to find a few videos specific to people with knee problems. For instance, he learned all about "chairobics," or aerobics practiced in a chair, which have given him some great no-stress activities to try while watching Matlock solve the mystery of the hobo in the bathtub with the missing kidneys.

#9. CONSIDER PHYSICAL THERAPY

George has always had good health insurance. As a result, he found himself a nice physical therapist, whom he jokingly refers to as his exclusive personal trainer. The YouTube videos were helpful, but his therapist has helped him better understand how to be mindful of things like posture and breathing while he practices safe, realistic exercises.

#10. VISUALIZE YOURSELF BURNING OFF STRESS AND OTHER NEGATIVE THINGS

Before George got moving, he didn't think he had many choices. Now, as he loses weight and gains some strength, he knows better. He feels good, and the image of him walking into his doctor's office, pointing his finger, and laughing in victory keeps him going. He's already up and out of the chair more than he thought possible, and all he can think about is what he wants to do next. He has sure showed them!

CHAPTER 7

RELEASE

When you're super stressed, every little thing gets to you.

Nothing particularly out of the ordinary was happening the day I exploded. The kids were being kids: jumping off furniture, knocking things over, breaking picture frames, fighting over the same toy, you name it. Then somebody drove down my road, and the dog started barking.

I was exhausted, at the end of my rope. I'd reached maximum capacity for noise and stimulation.

So, I started screaming at my children and my dog.

"Why are you being so immature?!" I yelled at the kids, with no sense of irony whatsoever. "And you," I said, turning my attentions on our dog, "why are you barking?!"

Suddenly I stopped, a little horrified at myself as the reality of the situation dawned on me. Nothing had gone wrong. The kids were being kids; the dog was being a dog. Realizing how ridiculous I was being, I burst out laughing.

SOMETIMES LIFE IS TOO MUCH

Everyone has had those times when life piles up and they're too exhausted to respond correctly. I was working two jobs, having the honor of taking care of a mother-in-law who was battling pancreatic cancer,[34] and trying to keep in touch with my friends—all while trying to be a good wife, mother, daughter, friend, doctor, and healthy person. I was trying to act like a superhero, but I'd forgotten to practice self-care and stress management along the way.

Being supermom, super wife, and super daughter-in-law each carry their own stress, but I was bringing plenty of stress home from work, too. My job carries a lot of responsibility. Some days, I'm walking out of a patient's room, wiping off a patient's blood from my shoes and tears

---

34   Unlike most sitcom characters who have contentious relationships with their mothers-in-law, I genuinely loved mine. We were always close, and the cancer brought us closer. She wasn't perfect—she was never on time a day in her life—but she was wonderful. When she saw me putting too much pressure on myself to be perfect, she would remind me that I was wonderful just the way I was. My life was better for having her in it, and I am grateful that I had the time, education, and capacity to be of service to her in her valiant battle against what would prove to be too formidable a foe. She handled it with grace and continues to inspire me every day. She is the "Bobbie" to whom this book is dedicated.

from my eyes, and telling his family that he didn't make it. Each loss and tragedy feels like a scar on my heart. When you've lived through enough of those moments, you realize your choices are to burn out, start drinking, or develop ninja-level, rock-star coping skills.

Since I didn't want to end up unemployed, in alcohol counseling, or in rehab, I chose to learn resilience. It's not always easy to admit when things are too much for me. If I admit that, it means I have to tell people I'm not perfect. And if I'm not perfect, does that mean that I'm not strong and that I can't do it all? I'm a doctor, dammit; I'm supposed to be a shining example of all that humanity has to offer! No pressure, right?

SNEAKY, SNEAKY

My blowup at my kids wasn't the first time stress had snuck up on me. I experienced constant stress during my medical residency, too. When you're a resident, you're working crazy hours. You aren't sleeping enough. You're trying to learn so much that they compare it to trying to drink from a fire hose. Sick people are everywhere. You spend half of the time certain you don't know how the hell to treat anyone.

I remember seeing a lot of people knitting around this time. When I asked what all the fuss was about, they all said the same thing, "Oh, this is great stress relief. You should try it!"

Since I'm good with my hands, I figured I'd give it a whirl. Should be easy, right?

Wrong. One day, my mother was watching me attempt to knit a blanket...I mean, a potholder. I was furiously white-knuckling the needles, clenching my jaw as I tried to get through the pattern.

"What are you doing?" she asked.

"Relaxing!" I snapped back.

Just maybe, knitting wasn't a good fit for me. I was happy to quit.

ASKING FOR HELP ISN'T EASY

On the road to becoming a doctor, I realized that education doesn't buffer you from stress. Just because I'm aware of a disease doesn't mean it's not going to happen to me. I'm aware of appendicitis, but it didn't protect me from getting it. I'm aware of the dangers of overexertion, but that didn't protect me from injuring a disc in my back. I'm aware of stress, but it didn't protect me from snapping at my dog and my kids.

Now, when patients come into the emergency department at the end of their rope, the first thing I do is congratulate them for coming in, for showing the strength to ask for help. Anybody can hide and deny, but true strength is helping yourself by asking for help from others and committing to getting stronger and healthier.

Asking for help isn't easy. We want to numb out, watch TV, dive into a cake, drink ourselves into the floor, or seek comfort in all the wrong places. We try so many unhealthy ways to take away the pain and stress that it's nothing less than a small miracle when we show the courage to actually admit something is wrong and we need help. When we do admit it, it's important to recognize and reward those moments, because this cultural belief that remaining stoic in the face of overwhelming stress is completely unrealistic. Nobody can maintain that forever.

WHY WE NEED TO DE-STRESS

Before I yelled at my kids and my dog on that fateful morning, if someone had asked me if I was stressed, I probably would have said, "No, of course not. I've got everything under control. Everything's fine." Sure, some things might have been bothering me, but I didn't think any of it was valid enough to get worked up about.

The thing is, your body doesn't care whether you are willing to admit that your stress is real or not. Your body still feels it and experiences its effects because it's beautifully and exquisitely designed to keep you alive. To accomplish this, you have this incredibly well-developed stress response system, which is commonly referred to as the fight, flight, or freeze response. When it's triggered, your heart rate quickens, your stomach starts doing somersaults, and you feel general nervousness from head to toe.

This process is exhausting and it unnaturally ages your body. When you're stressed, your cortisol system kicks in, which is designed to retain any available calories to protect and pad your body from hard times. This causes you to crave unhealthy food—fries, burgers, and other fatty and salty things your body thinks will help you survive war or famine. In stress mode, your body becomes completely focused on saving your ass, not caring how your ass looks in your favorite yoga pants.

Stress also raises adrenaline, making it more difficult to sleep. It's like having a pot of coffee right before bedtime. Both the cortisol and adrenaline processes could be useful in situations where there's actually a threat, but if we're not burning off these hormones through exercise, then it ends up doing a lot more harm than good.

NERD ALERT: HOW CAN YOU
TELL IF YOU'RE STRESSED?

It's hard to tell when you're stressed. I know all about the biochemical processes of stress and how they manifest, and yet even I used to have trouble telling when I was actually stressed or not!

One good way to tell whether you're stressed is if you have physical issues that your doctor can't find a basis for, including:

- Nervous stomach
- Frequent stomach aches
- Irritable bowels
- Shakiness
- Difficulty relaxing and going to sleep
- Chest pain or tightness
- Rapid breathing or difficulty catching your breath
- Headaches
- Jaw pain (from clenching or grinding teeth)
- Excessive fatigue
- Tightness in neck and shoulders (from defensive posture of holding shoulders up)
- Nausea or decreased appetite
- Restlessness
- Skin crawling feeling

The signs of stress can also manifest emotionally in the following ways:

- Anger and overreaction
- Decreased interest in things you normally enjoy
- Constant fantasies about winning the lottery or running away

To put it another way, if you're usually a big concert fan, but even the mere thought of going to a show suddenly makes you feel exhausted, overwhelmed, or nervous, there's a good chance you're stressed out. Recognizing some of these signs might help you realize there's something going on inside your body that you weren't aware of.

SURVIVAL MODE SHOULDN'T BE A FULL-TIME JOB

"I've got ninety-nine problems, and eighty-six of them are completely made-up scenarios in my head that I'm stressing about for absolutely no logical reason."

When you experience frequent stress, your body is in full-on survival mode. You start craving more carbs and fat because your cortisol system demands it. It thinks it's protecting you from famine, and in the short term, it is. However, in the long term, that constant supply of fatty, salty foods your body is demanding puts you at risk for a bunch of other diseases.

Your job when dealing with stress is to tell the body that the stressor has gone. The best ways to do that are through moderate exercise, stress relief, mindfulness exercises, adequate sleep, and all forms of self-care.[35] You may want to have the best butt on the block, but you won't get there until your body knows it's out of danger and doesn't have to be in fight-or-flight mode.

Unfortunately, most of us default to stress. We worry about all the bad things that are happening, the bad things that could happen, and the bad things that already happened in the past. Your body wants to help you, but it can't interpret these thoughts. It can't distinguish between an idea and reality. Your body believes what you tell it. And if all you're saying is, "Hey, body, shit's getting scary. Better activate survival mode," then you risk a whole range of long-term health problems. To meet your goal of being a healthy person, you have to start sending your body the right messages.

---

35   Note: Self-care isn't selfish! You can't bear the weight of the world with a broken back. My dear friend Joe Polish is great at reminding me that I can't fix the world with broken hands. I love giving talks on resilience, and he is a shining example of overcoming an abusive past, and drug and behavior addictions, and becoming an extraordinary success. If you haven't heard of him, you should search him out on Google, YouTube, and social media!

NERD ALERT: STRESS (OR A BROKEN HEART) CAN LITERALLY KILL YOU

You can literally die from a broken heart. The phenomenon, called Takotsubo's Disease, affects more people than researchers originally suspected. If you already have chronic, poorly managed stress and then are forced to endure an acute stressor like the death of a loved one, you face an increased risk of suffering, and possibly dying, from Takotsubo's.

Imagine a moment of intense grief—the death of a loved one, losing your home, or a huge emotional blowout with your spouse, for instance. The adrenaline and stress response can become so severe that it causes an actual heart attack. You feel chest pain, shortness of breath, maybe nausea, and sweating. You rush to the ER, and your EKG confirms that, yup, you just had a heart attack. The cardiologists rush you to the catheterization lab (where patients go to get angioplasty, stents, etc.) only to find out that your arteries aren't blocked enough to bring about a cardiac event.

Despite the seemingly mysterious cause, the damage can be just as severe, even leading to heart failure. Your heart pumping function is measured by what is called "ejection fraction," that is, how much blood is pushed out to your body with each pump. While normal is around 65 percent (weird, you'd think it would be nearly 100 percent, right?), after Takotsubo's, it can drop to 20 percent or lower. This means that your body isn't getting nearly as much oxygen-rich blood as it is used to, and all of your organs quickly start to feel the effects—from your brain to your kidneys to your lungs. You can't tolerate exertion and feel foggy and fatigued.

If you survive this initial attack, you will most likely recover to your normal function. That said, while Takotsubo's is survivable, it's best to avoid it altogether with good stress-management skills!

HERE'S HOW YOU HABIT THAT

Stress can be scary and hard to understand. What are the remedies? What can we do? For regular people like you starting with everyday resources (i.e., not millions of dollars, unlimited free time, a personal masseuse, etc.), the good news is that you have plenty of de-stressing remedies right in front of you.

ACKNOWLEDGE IT

"Relax. We're all crazy. It's not a competition."

The first step to addressing stress is admitting when you're feeling it. If I'm super stressed, I feel it in my stomach. You might feel it in your chest, in the way you're breathing, or in your clenched jaw, tight muscles, or even as a restless feeling in your hands and feet.

However you feel it, it's important to validate it. Acknowledge your stress and then find a way to share your difficulty with someone who can help you with coping strategies. The more coping strategies you build, the more resilient you'll be the next time a stressor appears.

To be sure, the next stressor *will* appear. You can't avoid your stress, pretend it's not there, or try to mask it with TV, bad food, drugs, or other unhealthy choices. You can't hide stress from your own body. If you try, it will manifest those problems physically.

BUILD COPING SKILLS

"It takes a remarkable person to enter the pain of a stranger."

I have a stressful job, but I'm just one of many, many people who can say that. In fact, through my work, I come into contact daily with others who are just as stressed out as I am—often more so.

I'm not their primary care doctor, they don't have a relationship with me, and yet, I'm the stranger charged with seeing them through the worst day of their life. I need to be available and present in the moment so they can open up to me.

I have seen the horrible things that people do to each

other. I have seen what different kinds of accidents or attacks can do to the human body. I have had to tell people that their baby has died, or that they have cancer. I can still hear the horrific screams of one particular burn patient sometimes when I sleep. This is the life I chose, but it *is* stressful.

I'm not saying other jobs aren't stressful. I'm not diminishing anything you or anyone else does. I can't imagine some other people's stressors—putting together huge business deals, creating technological advances, struggling to put food on the table, or wondering if they can afford insurance this month. Everybody experiences stress, and nobody's stress is better or worse. Whatever we experience, we have to learn from it in order to develop rock-star, ninja-level coping skills.

However, we live in a culture where it's not okay to admit when we're stressed. This is silly. There's no trophy for being the most stressed. We all want others to think we have our shit together, but the big secret of adulthood is we're all just making it up as we go and hoping no one else notices.

Acknowledging this universal truth is a big part of learning how to cope. It's not about comparing others' stress with yours. Rather, it's about understanding that we're all going through it, whether we're taking care of elderly parents with feeding tubes and twenty-four-hour needs or dealing with a flat tire. The more we acknowledge and validate others' stress, the more we understand our own and can begin coping.

CONNECT

With the birth of my first child, I experienced rather severe postpartum depression. It was uncomfortable talking about, since, as a new mother, I was expected to be filled with joy and wonder after the baby's birth. Make no mistake, I *was* overjoyed by the birth of my first child, but that didn't stop all the other negative feelings from creeping in and making me feel like a failure. It was such a difficult pregnancy that I had become emotionally exhausted. Add that to the exhaustion of caring for an underweight newborn, and the toll it took was real.

At first, I isolated myself. I didn't want anyone to know how I was feeling. I couldn't admit that, gasp, every single moment of my life and motherhood wasn't magically filled with unicorn dust and rainbows. Eventually, I told someone—and lo and behold, I didn't burst into flames! So I told a few more. When I finally decided to hold my head up and share my feelings, I was floored by the number of women who spoke up with me and shared their own experiences with postpartum depression.

I have found this to be true over and over. When people reveal that they have struggled with infertility, miscarriages, the loss of children, job loss, addiction, and any of their private woes, they find that they are not alone! Other people have been there, too! And by reaching out and connecting, we don't have to carry the burden alone.

For many of us, one of the best things we can do to address deep stress is to look up and connect with others. All it takes is for one person to open up that conversation, and all of a sudden everybody realizes it is okay to talk about it. The stress might not disappear, but through the sense of connection, support, and community you experience, you begin to realize there's nothing wrong with you. You're not broken. You're not a freak. You're not crazy or weak. You are a human being, and being a human being is often hard.

Connection can happen in the unlikeliest places. I had the privilege of attending the Genius Network Annual Event in Phoenix, Arizona. Considering this event cost $10,000 per ticket, you can imagine the caliber of content and expertise in the room. The Genius Network leader, Joe Polish, spoke candidly about his struggles with addiction as a way of dealing with his lonely and abusive childhood. This is not something that you would normally hear at a high-end business conference. Yet the effect on the conference attendees was profound. His talk gave comfort and social permission, and his openness elicited the same reaction in the crowd. Other people began sharing intimate feelings, allowing themselves to become so vulnerable that a few people broke down in tears. It was a remarkable and meaningful experience. The value delivered in content and connection made the ticket price seem minor in comparison.

After sharing his story, Joe explained how connection is the opposite of addiction. I think that applies to other painful situations as well, whether the issue is substance abuse, an abusive childhood, postpartum depression, miscarriage, relationship woes, job insecurity, or the many other kinds of stress and anxiety we all face. Connection is the opposite of depression, pain, and loneliness.[36]

MANAGING STRESS THROUGH DAILY ROUTINES

Awareness, empathy, and connection are all incredibly effective strategies for addressing and alleviating stress.

---

36 Joe Polish has a lot of other great thoughts about addiction and unhealthy behaviors as a response to stressors. Having suffered abuse as a child and feeling shy and disconnected, he turned to drugs in his teens. Today, he discusses the ways in which people treat addiction as a solution—not a good one, but a solution to pain and stress nonetheless. He taught me, "Instead of asking why the addiction, ask why the pain." Although he is a marketing guru and founder of the high-level mastermind groups Genius Network and GeniusX, he dedicates his time and resources to helping change the global conversation about how we view and treat addiction. He coauthored a book with best-selling author Anna David (herself a recovering addict and a shining light for those in need) and best-selling author Hal Elrod called *The Miracle Morning for Addiction and Recovery*. He also founded GeniusRecovery.com. If you or any of your loved ones are struggling with addiction as a way to treat your pain, I urge you to seek help. It is never too late! If a dead-broke carpet cleaner can clean up his act from addict to millionaire, you can too!

But what about everyday strategies, those little tricks you can use anywhere to help you calm down and refocus? That's what this section is all about.

RECOGNIZE AND REFRAME

"Not many people know this, but your car has a secret device on it called an 'indicator.' If you look at your steering column, you'll find a secret stick, which will activate a flashing light on the outside of your car. It flashes to let other drivers know in which direction you are thinking of going."

My commute to work used to trigger me into a big stress spiral. I thought all the other drivers were idiots. Nobody used their blinkers. Seriously, how hard is it to use a freaking blinker?! People cut me off. People were texting instead of paying attention to their damn driving! Eventually, I realized what this commute was doing to my mood and overall well-being, day in and day out.

I was in need of some serious reframing—a process where you take an event, in my case, being cut off in traffic, and choose to look at it in a different way. Sure, you could tell yourself the person who cut you off might be a colossal jerk whose only goal in life is to ruin your day. But what if you didn't make it about you at all? What if that person was rushing to the hospital to see a loved one who just suffered a severe trauma and wasn't expected to survive?

From that perspective, the traffic offender was simply a sad and stressed human trying to be there for their loved one's last breath. Now how do you feel about being cut off? Understanding? Sympathetic?

Unless you follow the person who cut you off to ask their story (and please don't do this!), you will never know the answer. So you can choose to feel angry and stressed with the "jerk" scenario, or you can choose to reframe it and send kind thoughts to the person who must be desperate to get somewhere. Either way, you have to slam on your brakes, but don't forget that only you have the power to slam the brakes on your bad attitude.

I enjoy my commute these days because I've changed my attitude toward it. I don't personalize other drivers' mistakes or aggressions. I let them deal with their own days so I can deal with mine. Now, I listen to audiobooks or sing along (loudly and slightly off-key) to my favorite tunes. I'm a rock star, party of one—and I don't even turn it down at stop lights! Judge me all you want; I'm having a great time. I changed my own habit and improved my day by recognizing and removing a stressful trigger.

BREATHING

You can alter your physiology and improve your health

simply by changing the way you breathe. To show you what I mean, I have a breathing activity to teach you.

Imagine something fearful, like bombs exploding in wartime or the agony of running uphill carrying a heavy load. Now, start taking quick, shallow breaths. Do this for about three minutes until you become hyperventilated. You'll start to experience the pH changes and other accompanying physiological effects as you blow off too much carbon dioxide. It will feel terrible. Your fingers might feel tingly, your face and lips might get a bit numb, and your hands and legs will start to cramp severely if you let it go on long enough. That's what a panic attack can feel like. I understand why people who are deep in the throes of this come to the ER; they feel like they are dying.[37]

Now that you've experienced some discomfort and learned how to recognize this feeling, it's time to experience the power of simple breathing techniques. To get started, sit comfortably or lie down. Pull your shoulders back if you're sitting, and let your chest open up. Place one hand on the top of your chest and one hand on your belly. Now take a slow, deep breath at your own pace. Take another deep breath and imagine pushing both

---

37 Note: If you did this exercise, it is important to return your breathing and carbon dioxide levels to normal. Take slow, deep breaths and remind yourself that the panic isn't real. This was only a test—and you passed!

hands out to fill your lungs. Take in a full-capacity breath, and then let it out.

Another variation of this is what's called the "square breathing" technique. Breathe in to a count of four, hold for four, exhale for four, hold again for four, and repeat. You can do this anywhere and people won't notice that you're doing it. I've used square breathing in staff meetings, with patients, or when my kids are painting themselves and the dog purple (seriously, parenting should come with more trophies).

Through these slow, deep breaths, you're telling your body, "This is the state that we are in right now." Do this for a little bit, and it triggers a substantial physiologic change, flipping the switch from fight-or-flight (the sympathetic nervous system) to rest-and-digest (the parasympathetic nervous system).

NERD ALERT: SYMPATHETIC VERSUS PARASYMPATHETIC NERVOUS SYSTEM RESPONSES

Your body has two opposing responses—the sympathetic fight, flight, or flee response, and the parasympathetic rest and digest relaxed response. They each serve important functions. You have the power to control your state by telling your brain how to feel. For example, when you are running from a bear, this is no time to try to digest your sandwich. Digestion shunts blood away from your running muscles. When you are under a big stressor, like being chased by a bear, the blood is shunted from your intestines to your muscles so you have the power to run or put up a good fight. This is why chronic stress can lead to digestion issues. And think of other things your body won't want to concentrate on when fleeing—building muscle, burning fat, increasing your libido and sexual desire, and cleaning up your arteries.

By the way, don't let the names fool you, they have nothing to do with "sympathy." It's just what some science nerd back in the day decided they should be called.

THE PARASYMPATHETIC VERSUS SYMPATHETIC SYSTEMS

Effect on organ	Sympathetic (fight, flight, freeze)	Parasympathetic (rest and digest)
Eyes	Dilates pupils (take in maximum light to evade threats)	Pupils constrict
Mouth	Decreases saliva (Ever felt your mouth go dry when you were stressed?)	Increases saliva (good for digestion)
Heart rate	Fast (Gotta be ready for that saber-toothed tiger!)	Slow
GI system	Inhibits digestion (Don't care about digesting your taco if you are fighting for your life! However, long-term residing in the stressed sympathetic state will give you indigestion and irritable bowels.)	Stimulates digestion
Bladder	Inhibits urination (Don't want to stop for a pee break on the run. Long term, not great for your bladder.)	Promotes urination (aaaahhhh!)
Adrenal glands	Stimulates release of adrenaline	Get to chill
Overall	Stimulated, tense, alert; functions not critical to immediate survival shut down	Calm, restoration, long-term survival

THE OPEN PALMS TECHNIQUE

Another method for turning your attention to your stress load is to open the palms of your hands into the shape of a book. Imagine that the pages of this book are filled with everything that stresses you out, whether real or imagined. Now, put this book (your hands) lightly against your face. How well can you see the world around you? How well can you see everything you love about your life and their endless possibilities? How well can you see the solutions to your stressors? Not very well, right?

However, when you move your palms just a few inches away, you start seeing the light and everything else around you. Your stress is still your primary field of vision, but you are at least able to see possibilities in the periphery. Slowly, move your hands farther away from your face until they are at arm's length. Has the stress gone away? Nope, it's still written on your hands. However, your perspective has changed. You can look up and see hope. Now you have a wider field of vision that allows you to start looking for ideas and solutions.

Sometimes, you just need to put your hands over your face, cry, scream, take a few deep breaths, and get a change of perspective. I use the open palms technique frequently because it reminds me in a tangible, physical way how focusing on my problems prevents me from discovering solutions.

MEDITATION

Meditation is tough. I already told you earlier that I'm still not very good at it. But then again, most of us aren't. Monks train full-time for years to be good at meditation. Just like I shouldn't be surprised that Lebron is going to dunk on me when I'm not practicing basketball (okay, he'd probably dunk on me no matter how much I practiced), I shouldn't be surprised if meditation isn't immediately yielding monk-like results on my first try—or even my twentieth.

For real, clearing your brain is difficult! I was focusing so hard on clearing my brain that when a thought would come in, I would be stressed that I was thinking when I was supposed to be clearing, dammit! Then I would think about thinking, and then I would think about how circular it was. Then I would think about the huge pile of laundry waiting, whether I'd remembered my daughter's permission slip, and why don't we know if there is life on other planets and...oops, there I go again. Ugh! Eventually, I realized that my mind will never be clear. Neither will yours! Mediation isn't about an *empty* mind, but rather a *focused* mind. It is about focusing on something specific. Whether it is a mantra, a fantasy, or a goal, the goal of meditation is simply to focus.

Before I understood what meditation really was, I complained to a particularly good meditation instructor that I found meditation nearly impossible.[38] She smiled and

---

38 Seriously, if you need a world-class meditation instructor, look up Julie Gandolf at Wave of Bliss meditation (www.waveofblissmeditation.com)—and tell her I sent you! Her calm and wise presence always makes me feel centered. And her retreats are legendary!

patiently explained said that while we may feel uncomfortable at first and may think it's impossible to stop our "monkey minds" from chattering away, meditation is highly effective for cleaning up old, accumulated stress. The trick is to keep practicing it and trust that you'll get better in time.

She also stressed the importance of finding something that works for you. You don't need to meditate in the lotus position. There are plenty of other forms of meditation that you may find more enjoyable. The goal is to put yourself in a space where you're not overthinking and worrying. Here are a few suggestions I like:

- Picture a trunk that holds all your old stressors, dating back to your first memories. Open it up, and put the day's stress inside. By making this a regular practice, you're not only shaking off the stress of that day and finding somewhere to put it, but you're giving yourself an opportunity to let a little bit of old stress out.
- Or you can use my newer more positive version of the trunk exercise. Imagine putting all of the awesome things about today into a big, beautifully decorated trunk. From the way the sun shone through the clouds, to the funny text you got, to the compliment from a friend, it is a place to store all of your wins in a safe place so you can take them out anytime you need an extra boost of sunshine.

- Download a guided meditation app. Find a pleasing voice that allows you to focus on their words, listen to the music, and follow along. Many of these apps are designed around progressive guided meditation techniques that take you through a series of relaxation messages to help you unwind your physical tension.
- Exercise, whether it's walking, jogging, or lifting weights, can put me in a meditative space.
- Practice yoga or swimming. Both require you to focus on your breathing and be mindful of your surroundings.
- Create a soundtrack for your life. Movies tell us how to feel by the background music. You always know when you should be feeling romantic or when the shark is about to sneak up and bite your butt. Make an energetic playlist for exercise, a mellow playlist for bedtime, or a stress-release playlist when you feel like you're at your wits' end.

Music is remarkably effective for altering your feelings and mindset. Use it to your advantage. Sing loudly in the car—or anywhere else where you aren't worried about people staring at you. Dance a little while you're at it. I also listen to podcasts, satellite radio, audiobooks, and a comedy channel. Remember to be flexible. Your preferences are likely to change both over time and throughout the course of the day.

If you only have five minutes of downtime, repeating your favorite mantra can be a great way of calming your mind and relieving stress. Just take a deep breath, say your mantra, and repeat. Here are three of my favorite mantras to help get you started.

- **"Resilience is a muscle!"** You aren't born with a fixed amount that gets used up. Everything you do toward self-care and stress management helps your resilience muscle get stronger and stronger. Make specific efforts to grow this, like a bodybuilder building biceps, so your resilience muscle is strong enough to bear the load of any stressor that comes your way.
- **"My brain is my bitch."** Your brain believes what you tell it. If you tell it that everything sucks and the sky is falling, it will believe you and oblige with the appropriate sympathetic response. If you tell your brain, "I've got this" and "Let's go bring on the awesomeness," it will believe you and give you the positive energy you need to conquer the world. Be mindful of this and take full advantage of your brainpower!
- **"Who am I not to?"** This mantra is the shortened version of a powerful quote by Marianne Williamson: "Our deepest fear is not that we are inadequate. Our deepest fear is that we are powerful beyond measure. It is our light, not our darkness that most frightens us. We ask ourselves, 'Who am I to be brilliant, gor-

geous, talented, and fabulous?' Actually, who are you not to be? Your playing small does not serve the world. There is nothing enlightened about shrinking so other people won't feel insecure around you. We are all meant to shine as children do. As we let our own light shine, we unanimously give other people permission to do the same. As we are liberated from our own fears, our presence automatically liberates others."

I use the "Who am I not to?" mantra all the time with patients wondering who they are to health up—and I used it for myself more than once while writing this book. But that particular mantra connects with me; yours might be different. Whatever mantra you choose, you need to hear it, see it, and say it frequently for your brain to absorb and fully integrate it. Repetition is the key to learning (remember me repeating that earlier in the book?). Write your mantra on a sticky note and put it on your desk, steering wheel, and refrigerator. Write it with a marker on your bathroom mirror. Say it at every stoplight. Use your mantra as your computer password so you are even typing it every day.

WHY REDUCING STRESS IS SO GOOD

When you make a daily habit of reducing stress, you're sending your mind a message that the world is safe and your body is okay. With any form of mindfulness, you help your brain get rid of the extra saddlebags dragging it down. Eventually, just like with regular exercise, you start to crave these little moments throughout the course of your day.

GOOD HABITS FEEL GOOD

Strangely enough, smoke breaks are a great example of how you can work stress relief practices into your daily life. Now, don't get me wrong. Smoking isn't good for you, not even a little bit. I'm definitely not encouraging you to take up or keep smoking.

However, the cigarette break is a commonly accepted ritual. It gives people the opportunity to take a break and step away from life's bullshit for a few minutes. In other words, tucked inside the bad habit of a smoke break is the good habit of putting life on pause for a few minutes and taking deep breaths. If you can replace smoking as the trigger, perhaps with taking a lap around the block or walking up and down the stairs, you can create a new healthy habit!

MINDSET SHIFT

It's up to you whether you look at moments in your life as obstacles or challenges. However, the more you practice stress relief and mindfulness, the more likely you'll be to greet anything that comes your way with determination and enthusiasm.

I was at a Genius Network event where hall-of-fame speaker Joel Weldon was discussing his positive-or-nothing approach to life. It didn't matter what terrible thing would happen; he'd trained himself to respond with "That's great!" no matter what. For instance, if his car just blew up, that was great, because now he had the chance to get a new vehicle. If he dropped $100 on the ground and it blew away before he could catch it, that was great because someone would get a wonderful surprise blown to them today.

I adore Joel and I admire his relentlessly positive approach to life. I'm pretty sunny, but he takes it to a whole new level of awesomeness. I'm not telling you to go that extreme. There are some things in life that I'll never find very great, and I'm sure you're the same way. I love the spirit of his message, though, and I've seen plenty of other motivational quotes that follow similar logic. Here are some of my favorites:[39]

---

39   The late, great Abraham Lincoln said it best: "Don't believe everything you read on the internet." Or, wait, maybe Benjamin Franklin said that. While I did my darnedest to find sources for these quotes, I often found them attributed to more than one person. If you read any of these and you know who actually said them, let me know!

- A diamond is just a piece of charcoal that handles stress really well.
- On the other side of your fear is everything you ever dreamed of.
- Attitude is the difference between an ordeal and an adventure.
- God never gives you anything more than you can handle.
- You have been assigned this mountain to show others it can be moved.
- The successful person is one who can build a firm foundation with the bricks that others have thrown at them.[40]

I have a few of these opportunity-minded quotes painted on my office walls. On one side is the Teddy Roosevelt quote, "Nothing worth having was ever achieved without effort." On the other, I have a quote from Vivian Greene, who said, "Life isn't about waiting for the storm to pass. It's learning to dance in the rain." This quote is probably why my kids and I put on our rain boots, grab umbrellas, and gleefully stomp in puddles on warm rainy days. My neighbors probably think we are crazy, but we are having too much fun to care.

Ultimately, the point is not to avoid or invalidate stress-

---

40 This quote is adapted from David Brinkley. His version was a little more targeted at men, but I wanted it to apply to everybody.

ors, but to greet them, process them, and get yourself toward a positive place. I'm not encouraging you to walk around saying, "Oh, life is fantastically full of rainbow sprinkles" in the middle of an earthquake. Instead, I'm saying there's real power in being able to face that earthquake head-on and see what you're made of.

THE DANGERS OF HOLDING ON TO STRESS

When you're not taking the opportunity to burn off stress, all those bottled-up feelings can cause a lot of damage. You know that feeling when you're in traffic, somebody stops suddenly, and you have to hit the brakes or you'll crash? Blood is shunted away from the GI tract and into the skeletal muscles, your heart rate and breathing quickens, your eyes dilate, and you become hypervigilant. That's your body in fight-or-flight mode. It's a useful response if you're running from a saber-toothed tiger or avoiding an accident, but if you're triggering it several times a day and doing nothing to alleviate it, then you've got problems.

STRESS ISN'T ONLY IN YOUR MIND

Your body's stress response is designed to keep you alive. The first part of any stress response is usually pain. Think of the recoil you feel when you put your hand on a hot stove. Your body doesn't like it, so it immediately tries to move you away from it.

Psychosomatics works the same way. When you feel stress indicators like achiness, fatigue, headache, chest pain, abdominal discomfort, or irritable bowels, that's your body trying to pull your mental hand away from the stress burner. Since you don't seem capable of addressing the problem yourself, it starts creating physical symptoms to get your attention.

These issues may have emotional triggers, but that doesn't make them any less real. Dying of a broken heart, for instance, isn't just a metaphor. The acute stress and grief you feel in this moment can absolutely lead to a heart attack and kill you. That's just one example, but unchecked stress can lead to all sorts of genuine health problems and diseases.

STUCK IN FIGHT-OR-FLIGHT MODE

Why does stress manifest itself physically in so many ways? The simple answer is it wants to protect you from danger. Unfortunately, it doesn't know the difference between a saber-toothed tiger and another reminder about a damn TPS report.[41] Modern stressors are rarely immediately life-threatening. Instead, they usually have something to do with work, life, and relationships.

Either way, when you experience stress, your adrena-

---

41 If you didn't laugh at this *Office Space* joke, then you probably have a case of the Mondays.

line and cortisol systems kick in—the same systems that cause so many problems when you're not getting enough sleep. If you were truly running from a saber-toothed tiger, you'd have a chance to burn these hormones off and return to baseline. In the modern world, however, our sedentary lives make this difficult. As a result, all those hormones keep kicking around in your body, making you feel like you drank an entire pot of coffee right before you went to sleep.

The stress cycle convinces your body that famine and war are imminent, so it decreases the functionality of your immune system and forces you to gain weight by storing every calorie it can get ahold of. At this point, your body is sending you constant messages to consume and self-medicate, which is why so many stressed people turn to overeating, distractions, drugs, and alcohol as bandages for stress. Unfortunately, these false stress-reducers don't actually address the issues and only lead to more long-term problems.

THE PERPETUAL CYCLE

The more you hold on to stress, the more your body encourages you to make unhealthy choices. And the more you make unhealthy choices, the more stressed you're likely to feel.

Over time, the constant barrage of fight-or-flight hormones begins increasing fatty plaques and stiffening your arteries, which are not meant to be exposed to big cortisol and adrenaline bursts every day. After several years of this, your arteries are like rusty kitchen pipes clogged with hair and grease.

Now you're more prone to high blood pressure, coronary artery disease, strokes, and kidney disease. One day, your body will try to send some blood through, as it normally does, but now your arteries are so clogged they can't handle the volume. In other words, don't let anybody tell you a problem is all in your head. Ignore stress long enough, and your body will pay the price.

NERD ALERT: THE UPSIDES OF STRESS

Stress is something that we usually give a negative connotation. But the truth is, stress isn't all bad! Some amount of stress keeps us engaged in a task, interested, and excited. If you were playing *Mario Kart* and all you had to do was drive straight—no obstacles, no blue shells, and no plummets off the track on Rainbow Road—it would be boring, right? We want ramps, jumps, and killer spins through fire to save the day! Overcoming a challenge gives a greater sense of satisfaction and accomplishment than completing boring or rote tasks.

Another upside of stress is improved strength. Our bones and muscles grow and get stronger under a stressor, such as lifting weights. If you never do a bicep curl, your muscles won't get very big. But every time you put that weight (stress) on the muscle, it grows.

Personal resilience can be the same way.

Recovering from a challenge or stress is resilience, like a deflated ball being reinflated back to its original shape. Strengthening your resilience muscles takes mental fortitude, specific skills, and practice.

Some exciting research has emerged in recent years in the field of posttraumatic growth or stress growth. People who experience trauma or stress don't just bounce back to who they were before the problem; they actually experience personal growth and positive change, becoming even better than they were before the stressor.

Think of the beautiful example of Malala Yousafzai, the young Pakistani girl advocating for education for girls and women when she was shot in the head by the Taliban at the tender age of fifteen. Remarkably, she survived. But she didn't *just* survive, she thrived. She was already an advocate, but after this incredible stressor, she became an international symbol of activism. She has founded a nonprofit, coauthored a memoir, and is the youngest Nobel Peace Prize laureate.

Talk about growth after stress! This isn't to say she didn't suffer and doesn't continue to struggle. It is that she was able to use the bad to create something positive.

You don't have to be shot (in fact, I discourage this!) to grow from stress. Imagine all of the things, big and small, in your life that stress you out. Getting your kids to school (or anywhere, if they are like mine!) on time, caring for an ill family member, struggling with past trauma, facing health scares, working in a difficult environment—it is not about what stressor gets the trophy for being the worst. It is about how *your* stressors affect *you*. You can choose how you react to them. You can learn to bounce back! And you can even learn to become better and stronger for having faced the stressor.

FINAL STRESS THOUGHTS

We're just about done with this chapter—and with the book! While we covered a lot about stress here, there's always more to learn. Generally speaking, whatever activity calms you down, helps you refocus, and puts you in the moment—that's a great way to blow off some steam.

Before we go, here's my big takeaway for you. It only takes five minutes to feel better. It's not about trying to fit an hour of yoga in every day. It could just be about singing your favorite song at the top of your lungs on the drive home. Stress release is a powerful tool for a healthy life, but if you don't Habit That activity, you won't get the benefit.

You can't think about broccoli and get healthier eating a doughnut. Similarly, you can't pay lip service to the value of meditation, mindfulness, and release without actually practicing it.

Finally, remember that you're not trying to avoid stress. That's impossible. Instead, your job is to greet the stressor, process it, and then habit yourself toward a more positive outcome. Start seeing the stress of your life as an opportunity to choose, learn, and practice healthy habits.

BILL LEARNS TO CHILL

Too much stress has already caught up with Bill once before, and he doesn't want that to happen again. He knows he has to change his lifestyle or risk another heart attack.

The problem is that Bill still has a million things going on as the head of his company. His doctor told him to consider meditation, and he gave it a half-assed try a couple times, but eventually gave up, convinced that hippie crap could never help calm his mind down. "What are they going to tell me next?" Bill says. "Do I have to grow a beard and a man-bun and start drinking kombucha?"

Despite his aversion to meditation, Bill is figuring out methods of stress relief that align with his idea of masculinity. He didn't really like yoga, but he did learn from step meditation that mental release doesn't have to be any of that so-called "hippie-Buddhist crap." He's also started to incorporate a power mantra to get ready for work and a relaxation mantra for his drive home.

Recently, he's started to investigate Tai Chi. He's heard it's all the rage in Japan, where top CEOs and high-level executives of some of his favorite companies are doing it. Bill sees Tai Chi's slow, deliberate movements as an appropriately masculine type of stress-relieving exercise—which is good, because after he overdid it at the gym recently and pulled a hamstring, his doctor isn't letting him do much else.

Bill also suspects his new Tai Chi practice will help with his global business deals. He's worked with some of these Japanese CEOs before, and if he can adopt some of their practices into his own business culture, he'll have created a great conversation starter.

As soon as he realizes this, the healthy living picture comes sharply into focus. Bill can adopt healthier practices and improve his business at the same time. Who knew?

BILL'S TOP TEN STRESS TIPS

Now, Bill is firing on all cylinders. Throwing himself into practice, he starts seeing that his concentration, focus, and mood are improving, too. This has forced him to acknowledge that his previous poor health wasn't just killing him, but was killing his productivity, too. These days, Bill finally understands that good health is also good business. To remind himself of the importance of managing his stress, he's come up with ten easy stress-releasing tips. Use Bill's ideas to health-up your own life!

#1. ELIMINATE NONESSENTIAL PEOPLE AND THINGS

Bill has become acutely aware of all the silly nonsense he's put up with in his life. Since his heart attack, he's taken stock of just about every person and thing in his life, asking himself whether they're making him happy and helping him move forward. He's already eliminated a few things—and a few people—and he's surprised at the weight that has lifted from his shoulders each time.

#2. MINIMIZE EXPOSURE TO UNAVOIDABLE STRESSORS

Bill has a vendor whom he considers, and I quote, "an epic-level douchebag." He can't stand the guy, but Bill depends on this man's service. One hour in the same room with him is like ten hours of being raked over hot coals. Bill can't avoid the guy entirely, but every time before they meet, he walks through his power mantra in order to calm his nerves and face the vendor on his terms.

#3. SCHEDULE SELF-CARE LIKE A MEETING

Bill already used his SMARTER Goals to schedule out his exercises. Now that he has accepted the benefits of mindful stress release, he's taking a similar systematic approach. He has times blocked out every day, he records his efforts, and he rewards his progress.

He's also learned to incorporate some of these wellness exercises into his family life. For instance, after dinner, he makes sure to take a short walk with his wife and kids. He sees this not as something he does in addition to dinner, but as something that's part of dinner. Now he feels more connected to his family and appreciates the extra chance to stretch his legs and take in some fresh air.

#4. FIND WAYS TO KEEP PERSPECTIVE

Bill hates the term *first-world problems*. Sure, his issues aren't on the same level as genocide and famine, but that doesn't mean his problems aren't important. If something is nagging at him, he's learned not to minimize, underestimate, or dismiss his feelings.

Acknowledging these annoyances has allowed him to put things in better perspective. Yes, he may have to deal with the insufferable vendor on Thursday, but on the bright side, he's regaining his health and has a fun family event planned for the weekend. By allowing himself to pull his hands away from his face (remember the open palms technique from earlier in the chapter?), he can acknowledge his problems without losing sight of all the other great things in his life.

#5. DAILY GRATITUDE

Since he started putting things in perspective, Bill has also discovered the value of gratitude. At first, he thought it was wishy-washy nonsense, but after trying it, Bill has seen a dramatic improvement in his mood. He realizes that there is no such thing as a self-made man, and that by being grateful to the people who have helped him become who he is, it strengthens rather than diminishes him. When he focuses on his love and appreciation for his family, inner circle, and business, he stops feeling like a grouchy asshole all the time.

To help reinforce this habit, Bill also practices this at dinner with his kids. As the family eats, they share what they were grateful for that day. Sometimes it's something silly like hopping, and sometimes it's something more serious, like the time they spent with their grandmother.

#6. BE AWARE OF OTHERS' ENERGY

Whenever Bill's sister calls him up, he ends the call feeling grouchy and edgy, and he's not sure why. This is usually when he and his wife start to bicker, though she's learned to defuse the situation by asking, "Have you been talking with Megan again?" That usually defuses the situation.

Bill is a little more aware of these things now. He loves his sister and wants to support her if she needs to vent, but she's an energy vampire and these conversations have a way of sucking the energy right out of him. To counter that, now when he gets off the phone with her, he takes a few calming breaths to center himself before rejoining his family.

#7. RECOGNIZE YOUR OWN STRESS SCALE POINT

Becoming more aware of his sister's energy has helped Bill tune into his own body's cues. Every day to start work, he asks himself where his stress level is on a scale of one to ten. Then he asks where different parts of his body are carrying that load on the same scale. Ones or twos he considers a normal day. Fives and sixes are worth noting, but manageable. Anything higher, and he knows he needs to address the problem right away.

#8. HAVE DIFFERENT ACTIVITIES FOR DIFFERENT TYPES OF STRESS RELIEF

Once Bill realized that you can release stress in a lot more ways than meditation, he started to build his toolbox. Sometimes, he just needs to sit still and be quiet. Other times, he needs to focus his body on something like Tai Chi. Sometimes, the best thing he can do is go to the gym and whack the punching bag. He matches the stress relief to his stressor.

He's even discovered what he calls "dish therapy." Bill has come to accept that sometimes he's going to be ragingly pissed off, and looking up pictures of fuzzy bunnies simply won't do. He needs to break something—now—and that's okay. Bill keeps a supply of thrift-store dishes in the garage. When the mood is right, he'll go in there, put on some safety goggles, and throw them as hard as he can against a designated wall. It's safe, he's not harming himself or others, and it always puts a big smile on his face.

#9. STAY CENTERED

When someone first suggested that Bill try different scents to calm and center him, he dismissed it as some silly froufrou crap. But then he realized he could choose whatever scent he wanted. His calming scent could be as macho as used motor oil if he wanted it to be.

Bill didn't end up choosing the motor oil, but he's always liked the smell of old books, and he's always enjoyed reading at night. His wife may tease him, but now he always takes in a big noseful as he settles down into his nightly routine.

#10. DEVELOP A MANTRA

Bill remembers the day of his heart attack well. He remembers staggering to the bathroom and all the negative thoughts that ran through his head. It's an image he'd rather do without, so he's decided to reclaim the bathroom as a power-giving, affirming space.

Before every big meeting, Bill takes a moment to look himself in the mirror and say, "You've got this," and "Trust yourself." They're simple mantras, but they resonate with him.

Those aren't the only mantras he uses. He also has a "get pumped" mantra for his drive to work and a "you kicked ass today" mantra for his drive home. Throughout the day, he'll also tell himself things like "you're effective" or "you're getting shit done." To connect this habit with others, he's even started asking his employees what their mantra is for the day.

CONCLUSION

LOCATE YOUR BROKEN LEG

Congratulations, you're almost through the book! Before you go, though, let's return to the analogy of the table and its four legs.

Imagine everything you value in your life: your family, your relationships, your career, and your hobbies. All the most important things in your life are balanced on the top of a table. If one leg is unstable, you have a wobbly table. If two legs are unstable, some of those important things could start slipping off. If three or four legs are unstable, the whole table could come crashing down.

To keep everything on the table—that is, to be a healthy person—all four table legs must be solidly in place.

If they are, if your health is good and balanced, it's amazing what you can do. You feel more energetic, you feel happier, and you have less depression and anxiety, healthier blood pressure, and a stomach free of bellyaches.

Living healthy is much simpler than people think. It doesn't have to be super complicated. With four stable legs, you have the freedom to feel how you want to feel and live how you want to live.

Many of us try to make healthy choices, but we often miss the issue right in front of our face. For instance, maybe you meditate and do yoga regularly and think that should help you with the chronic fatigue and mood swings you've been experiencing. Your mindfulness practice certainly helps, but if you're also completely sleep-deprived, you probably aren't seeing the results you want.

If it's not stress and rest, maybe it's diet, exercise, and weight loss. Right now, you could be saying, "Dammit, I am eating healthy and exercising, and I'm still not losing weight!" If that's the case, your body is telling you food isn't the problem. Maybe your stress-fueled cortisol system is telling your body to store every calorie it takes in, even the ones from the kale smoothies.

WHAT'S YOUR WEAKEST LEG?

We can all use help figuring out our weakest leg, or the pillar of health we need to work on the most to address our underlying issues. Luckily, I've designed a handy quiz just for this purpose (see Appendix E).

As you work through the questionnaire, be honest. Your objective is to identify potential blind spots in your lifestyle so you can build new healthy habits. No one's judging you. In fact, no one else will even see these results except for you—not your spouse, your boss, the college admissions board, or your crush from high school.

Hopefully, you have at least a few A and B answers, but if you have Cs and Ds in there, too, don't sweat it; now you know where to focus your energy first![42]

START WHERE YOU'RE COMFORTABLE

Hopefully, that quiz helped you learn something about your own health habits and you're already formulating a plan for how to address your weakest leg. However, before you start filling out your next SMARTER Goals worksheet, I want to help take some of the pressure off.

You don't have to start with your worst area—that is, your

---

42 For a full answer key and detailed breakdown of the questions and what they mean, visit www. drhopehealth.com.

table's weakest leg—if that's too much for you right now. It's good that you've learned you need to manage stress, for instance, but if you feel like focusing more on exercise for now, you'll still get some stress-reducing benefits along the way.

Start where it feels right for you, feel that rush of empowerment from your new healthy habits, and then take it from there. This will help you build some self-awareness around the issue and find something that works for you. Take it from me, I tried knitting because I saw it work for other people, but it made me white-knuckle tense. It wasn't a stress reducer for me at all.

I wrote this book to help build healthy habits that can start benefitting you today. However, I understand that we all go at our own pace. Change when you're ready, and when you have the confidence to think that you can handle more, keep rolling those quick wins forward into bigger and better habits. You will start accruing the compound interest and grow healthier over time.

KEEP LOOKING FOR BLIND SPOTS

The Weakest Leg quiz should have helped you identify areas you may have been ignoring, but I encourage you to keep looking for areas you can improve. We all have blind spots and selective recall. For instance, I had a patient who swore she was a healthy eater. However, when she took the time to accurately record what she was eating, she was a little shocked to discover that her days were dotted with junk food that she had been selectively ignoring, like M&M's at a coworker's desk and other unplanned nibbles on the go. What she thought her diet looked like and what it actually looked like were not consistent with reality.

My patient didn't have to become health food obsessed to improve her eating, however. She just had to change her focus, become aware of her blind spots, and acknowledge that her weak table leg was her diet. When she chose to focus on that, she made big changes quickly.

SOME KEY REMINDERS AND TAKEAWAYS

Speaker and author Zig Ziglar once said, "Motivation isn't permanent, but neither is bathing." Joe Polish, another prominent speaker, said, "Amateurs wait for inspiration. Professionals do it with a headache."

So what exactly are they getting at? Here's how I interpret it. It's okay that you're not always going to feel super motivated. However, it's important not to wait for that burst of inspiration to get going. Often, the action follows the motivation: first you do the thing, and then you get the feeling afterward. Here are a few other reminders and takeaways to help you on your way.

YOU BELIEVE WHAT YOU SAY

One day, I wasn't feeling well, but I thought to myself, *I want to get this done so I can get on with the rest of my day.* It was a struggle to start, but by the time I was done, my headache was gone and I was excited to tackle the rest of my agenda. In that moment, I was the kind of professional Joe Polish talked about, and that quick win took me one step closer to being the healthy person I knew I could be.

When it comes down to it, you are the person you say you are. If you call yourself "the fat kid" or "the person with no self-control," you will develop habits to match that persona. That day, despite how I may have felt, I told myself I was a professional and a healthy person, and that mindset made all the difference in accomplishing my goals.

I have a friend who constantly claims he's a terrible sleeper. He says it almost like a mantra, and his body believes him. I tell myself that I'm not only a great sleeper, but that I have great sleep habits. It can be hard to follow my normal sleep routine when I come home at two in the morning from a busy ER shift and I am still wired from being "on" for so many hours. However, I still go through my pre-sleep rituals, such as turning the lights down, taking a warm shower, and finding my pleasant scents. That way, my body knows the shift is done, and it's time to chill.

GET OUT OF YOUR OWN WAY

It can be hard to keep going sometimes. Even this book was evidence of that. Like many authors, I had a major crisis of confidence during the writing process. But rather than give up, I looked at myself in the mirror and said, "You know this stuff. You have helped many people, and your message could help even more. You've got this."

Then, I reminded myself of all the reasons I was going to work hard and write an awesome book. I'm passionate about helping people and sharing information that changes their lives. I care about others' health, and I want others to care as much as I do. Luckily, my brain believed everything I told it—because my brain is my bitch—and I was able to keep going.

Sometimes we need to get out of our own way, and that applies to getting healthier. You might think you need specialized knowledge, equipment, or training, but healthy habits don't depend on any of that. Just start doing what makes you feel good, pick a small bit of knowledge to learn for the day, do the best you can (and push yourself: your best is better than you think it is!), and go from there. And remember to always keep your expectations ambitious but realistic. No one becomes unhealthy overnight, and no one becomes a healthy person in a day, either.

BALANCE YOUR TABLE

By focusing on the four pillars we discussed in this book, you'll start to put your table in balance. When that happens, you'll feel empowered in every area of your life, free to walk through doors you thought had closed on you long ago.

There are plenty of success stories of people who went from homeless to being millionaires. However, their success didn't happen overnight and neither will your new balanced table. But while there may be no such thing as a health lottery, if you work toward the goal of becoming a healthy person with a good Habit That lifestyle, things will incrementally get better and better. One day, you won't even recognize your former self.

In the introduction, I told you about a friend who had been healthy before her divorce but took years to find her equilibrium afterward. Eventually, she made it back to the gym three or four times a week, regained that balance, and reached her goals. Afterward, she refocused on her new life and created habits that helped her sustain those gains, because she knew that maintenance is much easier when you've done the work and know what it took to get there.

These days, she's happy. She's still working as a fantastic, loving, successful pediatrician, but now she has a side business—helping working moms—that grew from her newfound motivation and self-empowerment. Her former self would have found this impossible, but by taking care of herself first, she discovered a new passion that she didn't even know was there.

HONOR YOUR SMARTER GOALS

The hardest part is over. The next step is to put on those gym shoes!

To do this, it's important to participate in the activities laid out in this book—finding your *real why*, identifying obstacles and objections, creating SMARTER Goals, and identifying your weakest leg. Doing the work cements the activity in your mind. In fact, I encourage you to go old-school with pen and paper. This will allow your brain to process these activities better than it could if you just banged them out on the keyboard. Sit down and think about your answers. By extending that effort, you're telling yourself, "This is important enough for me to write down. This will help me stick to my goals."

Once you're ready to put these worksheets into action, remember that you start where you start and wherever you are now is a great start! Even one SMARTER Goal, one healthy habit at a time is fine if it keeps you from feeling overwhelmed and overworked and keeps you on the road toward owning your identity as a healthy person. Setting twenty goals and reaching none of them isn't impressive. However, setting one goal and actually following through with it *is*—and even that single change will make a huge difference in your life.

MAKE IT WORK FOR YOU

You don't need a running trainer or a meditation instructor if those aren't good fits. You don't have to get up at four in the morning to meditate if that's not a fit, either (although I highly recommend *The Miracle Morning* by Hal Elrod. It might just change your mind about the power of getting up early and starting your day right!). If you're struggling with an activity or if you feel like what you're doing is crazy, try something else. Hate jogging? Try swimming. Or dancing. Your goal, after all, is to create *sustainable* habits. If keeping it up is a chore or a bore, it's not going to work out for you long term.

Don't just make it work; make it real. When I plan my exercises out for the week, I look at my week's schedule and identify the things that have moved around, such as family, social, and even work obligations. When the rest of my life is in flux, my workouts have to be, too, so I create activities that are flexible and work with my life as it is right now. Planning a long workout on an already packed day isn't real. It won't happen. So why set myself up for failure when I'm on the fast track to success?

Sometimes, I look at my calendar and realize I can't get as many workouts in as I'd like. That's fine. Even five minutes a day is helpful. If I miss a day, that doesn't mean I quit exercising. If I eat a piece of cake, that doesn't mean I have to eat the rest. In the grand scheme of things, I am still a person committed to my health and that's what matters.

MAKE YOUR HABITS SOCIAL

The more you connect with a community, the easier your goals will seem, the easier it will be to honor your commitments, and the more support you will feel. Say your goals out loud, talk to others about what you're doing, and make dates with friends centered on healthy-minded activities.

We were not designed to be solitary beings. Social connection boosts your oxytocin and makes you feel good. Being a healthy person isn't something you have to do alone.

Here's one good tactic that worked for me. Send out a post on Facebook looking for an accountability partner. You'll be surprised at how many people come out of the woodwork who are equally driven to change. In fact, you'll find that others can't wait to help, because they know that helping you will benefit them in the process!

USE MANTRAS

Again, your brain believes what you say. Mantras don't have to be esoteric words from ancient texts. They just have to be things that resonate with who you are.

My mantra used to be long and cumbersome. It went something like this, "Oh no! I have a lot of stuff I have to do today and not very much time, and I have no idea how I'm going to do it all!" It wasn't very catchy, and it also didn't reflect the mindset of a healthy person.

Now, my mantra is simpler and much more affirming: "You've got this." It keeps my mind on what needs to get done in the moment. If I'm on a call, I focus on the call, not also checking my email and doing fifty other things. If I'm with a patient, I focus on the patient (which I'm sure my patients are glad to hear). When that's done, I go to the next thing. Whatever the day asks of me, I can handle it. I've got this.

Once you find a mantra you like (and I encourage you to come up with as many as you can), write it down so your brain processes it better. You should see how many things get written on my hand, my mirror, and on sticky notes and index cards (which eventually find their way to my car and my computer). I've even started changing my computer passwords to inspirational mantras to make them a more active part of my everyday life.

YOU'VE GOT THIS

Well, here you are now at the end. You've done what many people don't do: you got a book, opened it, and read it to the end! That says volumes about your own drive to become healthier. Something in this book spoke to you, and now the message belongs to you.

This book is just the conduit. *You* have the power. You are your own best hope. Only a small percentage of people who buy a book open it. A smaller percentage finish it. Even fewer start putting the changes into action.

To this smallest of small percentages, to the special and powerful readers who are truly ready for something new in their lives, I speak to you. You've found your *real why*. You have the power to achieve the change you crave. You. Are. Unstoppable!

KEEP IN TOUCH

That's it. You're all done with the book. Feels pretty good, doesn't it?

If you'd like to keep learning more about the Habit That lifestyle, you can join our Facebook community and engage with other like-minded, healthy, perfectly imperfect, and awesome people:

- The Habit That website: http://www.drhopehealth.com
- The Habit That Tribe on Facebook:[43] https://www.facebook.com/groups/1983040705045797

Thanks again for reading, and I look forward to connecting with you!

---

43 Admittedly, this is a bit of a cumbersome URL. Alternatively, you can just go to Facebook and search "Habit That Tribe." That should do the trick, too!

APPENDIX A

FIVE-MINUTE HEALTH-UPS

The following are some great activities that you can do to improve your health in each of the four pillars. Some might not resonate with you or fit your needs, while others may help change your life! I ask that you complete *each* exercise here to help create and strengthen your healthy pathways. All of the activities that help you, keep doing!

Many of the activities ask you to set a timer for five minutes. It is perfectly okay to go beyond this time if you are brimming with ideas! The plan is that you do them for at least five minutes, but you don't have to stop there if you don't want to.

BARRIER AWARE

In this activity, you will brainstorm every possible barrier you have to making healthy habit changes in your life. I want you to think of absolutely anything that can be an excuse, hindrance, deterrent, hang-up, limitation, obstacle, restriction, or hurdle. These should include current known barriers, such as time, old habits, knowledge gaps, etc. In addition, I want you to use your best pessimistic imagination and list things that could go wrong that you might have to overcome while working toward your goals. Things like breaking your ankle, car engine problems, a sick family member...that sort of thing.

Now that you have the mindset and intent of this exercise, grab a piece of paper or get to a blank document on your computer. You are doing this list-style. Don't edit, just mind-dump anything you can think of; there are *no* wrong answers! Set a timer for five minutes and go! (It is okay to go longer or return to this anytime if you think of or encounter any additional barriers.)

BARRIER BUSTING

In the Barrier Aware activity, you listed all the possible obstacles you do/might face on your road to becoming a healthy person. Now that you are aware of what might be holding you back, you are empowered! It is much easier to overcome a barrier with a plan. Use your list from the

Barrier Aware activity, and next to each barrier, write a way you can overcome or work around it to stay on your goal to being a healthy person. If the barrier is injury, for instance, what can you do if you can't do your usual exercise? This will get you in the habit of understanding roadblocks without being defeated by them!

EAT
MIND FRAME WORD LIST

Take out a sheet of paper and your favorite writing utensil or open a new document on your computer. Have a timer available. First, imagine that you are an unhealthy eater. Think of every word (e.g., *heavy*, *greasy*, *guilty pleasure*) you can that you associate with unhealthy foods—the risks, how they make you feel, and all of the bad qualities, etc. Set a timer for two-and-a-half minutes, and during that time, make a list of everything that comes into your mind.

Now start a new list. This time, think of every word (e.g., *light*, *nourishing*, *clean*) that you can associate with healthy foods—the benefits, how they make you feel, and all of the good qualities. Set a timer for two-and-a-half minutes, and during that time, make a list of everything that comes into your mind.

Keep your lists of words for healthy and unhealthy foods

near where you eat. Anytime you are not sure whether you should eat a food, see which list it fits on. And if you are tempted to eat something unhealthy, look at the list of healthy words. If it doesn't fit those things, don't eat it.

WRITE YOUR FOOD GOALS

Review your list of words that you created for healthy foods—words such as *wholesome*, *fresh*, *clean*, and *nourishing*. Foods that evoke this kind of vocabulary are the types that you should feed your body with. Now, let's write out some specific food goals. As we talked about, colorful, fresh, real foods give you the best health results. It is hard to get every food every day, so I'd like you to imagine you're eating a week at a time, rather than a day at a time. Want to get a serving of healthy leafy greens each day? Write a chart for the week with seven check boxes for leafy greens. Each time you eat a serving, give yourself a check! Your chart should include all of your important food goals you want to nourish your body with. Think number of servings of things such as berries, cruciferous vegetables, and healthy fats. Post it on your fridge so you see it each day. There are also a ton of food-tracking and goal-setting apps. Use your five minutes to create your chart or learn how to use your awesome new app.

WRITE A MEAL PLAN FOR THE WEEK

Do you find yourself grabbing convenience food on the go more often than you would prefer? Use this easy five-minute fix! You know what your schedule is for the week and where you will be. Why not plan your meals the same way? Here's how a few days of your list could look:

- **Monday.** Working late, no time to make something. Make your meal on Sunday and have it ready. Or, plan healthy takeout, such as sushi or one of those awesome make-your-own-salad places that are popping up everywhere now.
- **Tuesday.** Dinner with the family. Make sure you have the recipe you want to cook and all of the healthy ingredients on hand.
- **Wednesday.** Dinner out with friends. Look at the menu in advance and make a healthy selection. Order first so you won't be tempted by others.
- **Thursday.** Yay, tacos! You can health-up your taco with vegetables.

And so on. The more you plan your food in advance, the less you have to rely on chance (and low willpower states that lead to less-than-nutritious choices). By taking five minutes to plan out some or all of your meals for the week, not only will you decrease the likelihood of making spur-of-the-moment junk food decisions, but you'll also begin to form a new healthy habit!

CHOP AND CONTAINERIZE

Create your own convenience food. Choose a day to do this each week. The five minutes it takes will definitely help you health up! Chop up veggies and put them into grab-and-go containers in the fridge (consider reusable containers rather than disposables so you can health up the environment, too!). You can containerize serving sizes of fruit, nuts, hummus, and all kinds of healthy snacks.

CRAVING BUSTER AND BINGE-STOPPING EMPOWERMENT

Have you ever found yourself with a powerful craving for something unhealthy? Or found yourself staring intensely at the cake after already having had a piece (or two!) and feeling like you might eat the whole thing? Let's create a list together that you can keep handy in your kitchen or carry with you when you are out. You will have an entire arsenal of ideas to fight back when the craving monster hits.

Take out a sheet of paper and writing utensil or open a new document on your computer. Have a timer available. Set a timer for five minutes and write down as many ideas as you can for things you can do to snap yourself out of the crave cave. Here are some ideas to get you started. Write these on your list, and then add your own:

- Brush your teeth
- Eat a citrus fruit
- Go for a walk
- Set a timer and do jumping jacks or run in place
- Drink a big glass of water
- Call a supportive friend
- Write down your feelings

SLEEP

MIND FRAME WORD LIST

Take out a sheet of paper and writing utensil or open a new document on your computer. Have a timer available. First, imagine that you are sleep deprived. Missing sleep, skipping sleep, and feeling exhausted. Think of every word you can (e.g., *exhausted, ineffective, sluggish*) that you associate with this state of being—the risks, how you feel, and all of the bad things that can happen. Set a timer for two-and-a-half minutes, and during that time, make a list of everything that comes into your mind.

Now start a new list. This time, think of every word that you can associate with adequate amounts of high-quality sleep. The benefits, how you feel, and all of the good qualities. Set a timer for two-and-a-half minutes, and during that time, make a list of everything that comes into your mind (e.g., *refreshed, energized, chipper*).

Keep your lists of words for inadequate sleep and adequate sleep near your bed as a reminder of how good you feel when you get sleep and how awful you feel when you don't. When you are tempted to skip sleep to get other things done, review your lists and decide how you want to feel.

BEDTIME ROUTINE

Having a routine that you follow each night helps send your body the signal that it is time to go to sleep. Consider having a pleasant, relaxing scent that you associate with sleep, do a series of stretches, journal, think of things you are grateful for about your day—whatever feels right for you. The five-minute routine should be practiced nightly to help create a habit. Your room should be cool, dark, quiet, and free of electronics. You can do your routine before or after your hot shower/bath if this is also part of your wind-down routine. Create your routine and share your ideas with other like-minded people in the Habit That Tribe Facebook group.

PROGRESSIVE RELAXATION

When you are in your bed in your cool, dark, and quiet room ready for sleep, this is the time for this activity. Be done with everything else so you don't have to get out of bed or move much after this activity. It is designed to be the last thing you do before drifting off to good-quality sleep for the night. You can purchase tracks that narrate this for you or do the one written here.

Lie flat on your bed with arms down by your sides, take a deep breath in, and exhale. Now squeeze your toes tightly and in a whisper voice, count back "five, four, three, two, one, release." When you say "release," relax your toes. Now point your toes, extending your feet with good muscle effort and count back "five, four, three, two, one, release." This time, when you say "release," relax your feet. Now flex your feet up to your head and repeat the countdown and release.

Move upward through your body, squeezing and then relaxing muscles and joints in this pattern: straighten knees, squeeze legs, squeeze buttocks, tighten abdomen, squeeze hands, bend wrists, straighten elbows, shrug shoulders up, turn neck to the right, turn neck to the left, bring your chin to your chest, push your head into the pillow, squeeze your mouth shut, and lastly, squeeze your eyes shut for your last "five, four, three, two, one, release."

BURN

MIND FRAME WORD LIST

Take out a sheet of paper and writing utensil or open a new document on your computer. Have a timer available.

First, imagine that you are completely sedentary with no exercise or activity. Think of every word you can that you associate with this state of being—the risks, how you feel, and all of the bad things that can happen. Examples could include *tired*, *achy*, and *sluggish*. Set a timer for two-and-a-half minutes, and during that time, make a list of everything that comes into your mind.

Now start a new list. This time, think of every word that you can associate with healthy movement and adequate amounts of activity. The benefits, how you feel, and all of the good qualities (e.g., *strong*, *energized*, *flexible*). Set a timer for two-and-a-half minutes, and during that time, make a list of everything that comes into your mind.

Keep your lists of words for inactivity and quality activity as a reminder of how good you feel when you get moving and how awful you feel when you don't. When you are tempted to skip active movement for sluggish, sedentary activities, such as plopping in front of the TV or playing on your phone, review your lists and decide how you want to feel.

FIND YOUR BURN STYLE

If you don't already have a regular exercise routine, this will help you! There are some activities that will both resonate with you and are available for you to do. For instance, you might hate jogging but enjoy swimming. Find a pool that you can use for exercise, and schedule it into your week. If you want to jog but haven't started, spend the time finding a nearby route or trail. If you want to work out from home, look up YouTube videos that are targeted toward your fitness level and goals. It is worth the time you take to find something you like and will stick with. Just don't get sucked in to YouTube and spend hours watching animal videos—laughing is great medicine, but it doesn't count as exercise!

PLAN YOUR WEEK IN ADVANCE

Your exercise should be an appointment on your calendar and treated with the same importance as any other appointment (more important than getting your dry cleaning, for sure!). Sit down for five minutes each week and map out your exercise plan for the week. Some days are busier than others; make sure your plans are achievable. Even if you travel for work, you can schedule time at the hotel gym or take the time to search for places to work out at your destination.

THE "I ONLY HAVE FIVE MINUTES" FIVE-MINUTE WORKOUT

Get out that timer! First minute, do jumping jacks. Second minute, high knees (running in place, but with your knees higher. Third minute, burpees (YouTube a video if you don't know how to do these). Fourth minute, star jumps (like jumping jacks, but higher—YouTube can teach you). Fifth minute, lunges. I guarantee you will be breathing hard after this! It's okay to create your own five-minute versions; just make sure you are challenging yourself! Even on a busy day, you can carve out a quick five, right?

RELEASE

MIND FRAME WORD LIST

Take out a sheet of paper and writing utensil or open a new document on your computer. Have a timer available. First, imagine that you are completely stressed out. Think of every word you can that you associate with this state of being—the risks, how you feel, and all of the bad things that can happen. Examples could include *frazzled*, *exhausted*, and *out of it*. Set a timer for two-and-a-half minutes, and during that time, make a list of everything that comes into your mind.

Now start a new list. This time, think of every word that you can associate with finding ways to manage stressful things in your life—the benefits, how you feel, and all of the good qualities. Examples include *strong*, *empowered*, and *relaxed*. Set a timer for two-and-a-half minutes, and during that time, make a list of everything that comes into your mind.

Keep your lists of words for stress versus empowerment as a reminder of how good you feel when you manage your stress and how awful you feel when you don't. When you are tempted to skip stress-managing activities, review your lists and decide how you want to feel.

CREATE YOUR OWN SUPER WORLD

When you are stressed, down on yourself, or otherwise anxious, go to your Super World. Wherever you are, you can visit when you need a brain break. Choose things like colors and location, and imagine the sights, smells, sensations, and sounds in vivid detail. The only rules are that this is a place where only positive things can happen and you achieve what you set your mind to. No other rules are necessary, so unplug from reality and build your Super World however you want and visit whenever you need.

You are a hero here! Want to fly? No problem! Want to save cuddly animals from villains? Go for it! Want to teleport, have unlimited riches, and have your own tropical island? It's yours! Your Super World can evolve and change whenever you want it to, and it is only yours. When your day is hard and your mood is low, take a quick trip here, to a place where you are in control. When you are ready, take a deep breath and teleport home to reality with a superhero boost and face your next challenge stronger because you just saved the world from a shark-covered meteor (I'm sure this will be a movie soon). After such heroics, the rest of your day will be a piece of cake.

BREATHING EXERCISES

When you are stressed, taking a five-minute timeout can really help get you calm and out of fight-or-flight body physiology. Go somewhere that you can be alone (e.g., the car, a stairwell, your office) and start your timer. Get into a comfortable position and start square breathing: breathe in for four seconds, hold your breath for four seconds, breathe out for four seconds, and hold your breath for four seconds. Just breathe and count.

Some people like to imagine breathing in good things (energy, beauty, sparkles, happiness, confidence) and breathing out bad things (stress, fear, worry, anger). Building a five-minute timeout to breathe each day will go a long way toward helping your stress!

GUIDED MEDITATION

If you find that you can't clear your mind for meditation (don't worry, many people struggle with this!), find a meditation that occupies your mind in a productive and relaxing way. There are many guided meditations available as apps or MP3s, on iTunes, on Audible, and many other sources. Try out a few different ones to see what fits your needs best. Schedule it in your calendar as an appointment to increase your likelihood of keeping it, or pull out your guided meditation app anytime you need a stress-relief break. Get double duty by choosing a relaxing sleep-promoting one to use at bedtime to decrease stress and help you drift off into quality sleep.

WRITE A BURN LETTER

Take out a sheet of paper and writing utensil or open a new document on your computer. Have a timer available. Think of something or someone that upset, hurt, or wronged you in any way. Whether this person or event is in the recent or remote past, if you are still carrying strong feelings, write them out. Pick one topic or person at a time. Set a timer for five minutes and let your thoughts flow freely and write everything that comes to mind. Don't worry about sentence structure or grammar—this is a releasing exercise!

No words or ideas are off-limits. If you have more to say after five minutes, continue until you have it all out for the day. Plan on doing this for three to five days in a row (or as long as necessary!) until you get every possible feeling, thought, and impression about this person or event down on paper. Wait a few more days to see if anything else comes to mind. You can even repeat any of the thoughts on paper each day until the strength of the anger and hurt is lessened.

When you are ready (you will know when) and you are completely done with this specific person, event, or idea and have written all you have to say, it's time to burn. Whether you put the letter in the shredder, tear it up into the garbage, or actually burn it (please do this in a safe manner!), you need to destroy it. Release the pain and anger and hurt. Forgive, even if that person doesn't deserve it. The forgiveness is for *you*. If you find you have residual anger or hurt, write it out again and again and burn. The strength of the pain *will* diminish. There is no limit to how many times you can do this activity. Set aside five minutes as often as you can to write out your hurts. Also consider speaking to a licensed counselor if you feel that you are struggling with any of these feelings.

FIVE-MINUTES-PER-DAY GRATITUDE

Take out a sheet of paper and writing utensil or open a new document on your computer. Have a timer available. Write out everything that you love, things that make you happy, things and people you appreciate that have made the world and your life a better place. An additional exercise you can do with this is to spend your five minutes writing a letter to someone for whom you are grateful. Be verbose about the wonderfulness they have brought into your life. Imagine how great they will feel reading it!

FIVE-MINUTES-PER-DAY FRUSTRATIONS

You know those day-to-day frustrations? Maybe minor irritants (like autocorrect changing words you didn't want to change!), traffic jams, and a messy kitchen counter? On good days, the small things feel like small things. But when our stress level is higher, small things can feel like big problems.

If you find that you are grumpier than you would like to be, start a running log/journal to see what patterns emerge. Take out a sheet of paper and writing utensil or open a new document on your computer. Have a timer available. Set a timer for five minutes and write all of the things that bug you that day. If you have more left after the time is up, keep going until it's all out. Write the date on it. Commit to doing this at least three times per week or on any day that you have some annoyance and frustration.

After several sessions, see if you notice patterns—certain things that get your goat over and over. Once you figure out the little things that bug you big time, start to EMPTY (**E**liminate, **M**inimize contact with, **P**erspective, **T**hankfulness, **Y**ou time) your annoyances. Can you eliminate the thing from your day/life? Great! If not, can you minimize your exposure to them/it? Can you get perspective on the thing? (Traffic may be annoying, but you have a vehicle, gas money, places to go, working limbs to operate the vehicle—that kind of thing.) Prioritize addressing the problem constructively (listen to audiobooks in traffic jams, call loved ones using hands-free devices). Imagine how the problem could be worse, and be thankful that it isn't at that level. Then make some time for *you* to have positive activities in your life that are stronger and more frequent than the annoying things.

EMPTY the stress and tip the balance of your day toward more positivity. It is impossible to lead a completely stress-free life! Although you can't always change the things that stress you, you are empowered to change how you react to the stressors! EMPTY as many as you can!

APPENDIX B

THE 12 REASONS EXERCISE

THE 12 REASONS

You are ready to make healthy choices. You **want** to change your life and make a positive difference! Creating better habits is simple...*but it isn't always easy!*

" Motivation gets you started. Habit keeps you going. "

In order to make meaningful, lasting changes, you need to turn your behaviors into habits. We can't rely on the fickle tides of motivation for long term success. Motivation can be so fleeting! **Let's get in touch with your real 'WHY'.** This is that deep down true-blue reason you want to make healthy changes. For some people, it is fear of disease or disability, for others, it is about having control.

Some examples I've heard over the years:

- o I quit smoking because I didn't want to get wrinkles
- o I quit smoking because I heard second-hand smoking could give my dog cancer
- o I want to lose weight because 'that witch Heather' is skinnier than me and I can't let her win
- o I want to get in shape so I feel comfortable having sex with the lights on
- o I need to exercise more so I can play with my kids without being embarrassingly short of breath
- o I am going to change because I'm never going to be humiliated by getting my butt stuck in a chair ever again!

The reasons are as varied as the people making them. They don't have to be noble or world-changing, *they just have to be yours*. Whatever will truly help keep you on track when the going gets tough and you want to quit!

THE 12 REASONS

Write 12 reasons that you want to change your health for the better.

Yes, 12! The first few will be easy...avoid heart attacks, lower cholesterol, feel better etc. *But I want you to dig deeper.* This isn't the kind of thing you just tell your coworkers, doctor, and acquaintances. The real answer will be the one you hesitate to write down. The one you would cover up if you were writing in a classroom. It might be number 1 or number 12, you will know it when you feel it. The others matter too. These 12 reasons will be your guide, your North Star, on your journey to an empowered healthy life!

1. _____

2. _____

3. _____

4. _____

5. _____

6. _____

7. _____

8. _____

9. _____

10. _____

11. _____

12. _____

APPENDIX C

THE SMARTER GOALS WORKSHEET

Dr. Hope's SMARTER Goals Planner
Use SMARTER planning to achieve success!

Remember the overall goal: **be a healthy person.**
Now, let's break it down to make it happen, one goal at a time.

S	Specific	The more specific the goal, the better the chance for success. Instead of "I want to get in shape", make a goal to exercise 20 min per day. Break the goal into smaller pieces to make it manageable.
M	Motivation	Why do you want to achieve this particular goal? What will keep you going when it gets challenging. What is the final outcome you want and how can you stay on the road to get there?
A	Action plan	Use action-oriented statements – "I will ___". What are the steps you will need to achieve your goal. Plan time, equipment, support, location, etc. The less you leave to chance, the better your chance for success!
R	Roadblocks	Roadblocks will happen! People, time, and circumstances will make it more difficult to achieve your goal. List potential roadblocks that might occur (including waning motivation) and how you will overcome these roadblocks to reach your destination!
T	Time table	All goals should be grounded with an ambitious YET realistic time frame. You want to push yourself! What can you do today? This week? This month? This year?
E	Evaluate, Evolve, Excitement	How are you doing along the way toward your goal? As part of your action plan, make time to reassess. If your original goal was exercise 20 min per day and after a few weeks, you find it easy to do 30 min (or 3 stretches of 10 min), let your goal evolve. Approach your goal with enthusiasm, it is YOUR goal and you will reap the rewards of your excellent efforts!
R	Record and Reward	Write down your SMARTER action plan!! Writing it will give you substantially greater success than just thinking it. Keep it where you can see it, record your success. Plan rewards at certain milestones, you deserve it!

"A GOAL WITHOUT A PLAN IS A WISH!"

- Antoine de Saint-Exupery

Top Goal: I am a HEALTHY PERSON.

In order to be a HEALTHY PERSON, I am going to *(fill out the form below)* . I **know** I can achieve this by getting SMARTER.

Specific Goal

_____

Motivation

_____

Action Plan

_____

Roadblock

_____

Timetable

_____

Evaluate, Evolve, Excitement

_____

Record & Reward

_____

Post this somewhere you will see it daily! Each goal should have its own sheet.

APPENDIX D

TRACKING YOUR FITNESS GOALS

FITNESS GOALS

Work out 3 times per week (156 times/year) with rewards after you finish ten workouts. Pre-plan your fun rewards – a movie, a night out, new shoes – whatever helps keep you working toward your goal.

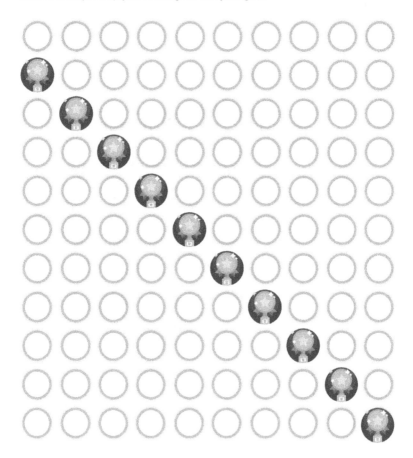

APPENDIX E

IDENTIFYING YOUR WEAKEST LEG

1. Have people told you that you look or seem tired?
   A. Rarely. I might be able to recall a few instances in the past few years.
   B. Now that you mention it, I have noticed people mentioning this.
   C. I'm definitely not enjoying the frequent comments about bags under my eyes and looking tired.
   D. Several people have expressed concern about this and wonder if I am okay.

2. How do you handle negative feedback from others?
   A. I usually take it in stride and see it as a chance to improve myself.
   B. It depends on the intent, how much I like the person giving it, and my mood that day.

C. I get defensive and argue about it.

D. I burst into tears or fits of anger.

3. How often do you crave junk food?

 A. On occasion, such as smelling popcorn at the movie theater or special holiday treats.

 B. A few times per week, especially when I'm tired or stressed.

 C. Like clockwork in the afternoons and evenings.

 D. Pretty constantly, if I'm honest.

4. How much caffeine do you consume, whether from coffee, tea, soda/pop, energy drinks, caffeine pills, etc.?

 A. I will enjoy a good cup of something now and then.

 B. Usually one per day, but I don't feel bad effects if I skip it.

 C. I drink multiple per day, and I get headaches or fatigue if I don't drink any.

 D. I am reaching for caffeine and stimulants daily to get through my day—can't go without it.

5. Describe your usual mood.

 A. I am generally upbeat and steady with the usual ups and downs of life.

 B. I've had times where I'm in a funk or overreact but nothing too concerning.

 C. I am noticing depression, anxiety, anger, or moodiness more often than calm and happiness.

 D. My moods are affecting my relationships and/or work and I feel labile.

6. You feel depression and anxiety...
    A. When something bad happens, like a death of a loved one.
    B. Periodically from time to time.
    C. More often than feelings of calm or happiness.
    D. Constantly. I feel like a mess.
7. Describe your memory and concentration.
    A. Pretty good, if I do say so myself.
    B. I occasionally forget names or where I put my keys, but I feel sharp.
    C. I feel foggy and have a hard time remembering things.
    D. I am forgetting important things, having trouble concentrating, and it is negatively affecting my life.
8. When I am driving...
    A. I enjoy the radio or listening to an interesting book or podcast.
    B. I am irritated with other drivers.
    C. I forget part of the drive and am surprised when I arrive, or I start driving to one destination rather than another (e.g., kids' school instead of work).
    D. I nod off frequently and have swerved multiple times from not concentrating.
9. When I wake up in the morning, I feel...
    A. Pretty good!
    B. Somewhat tired if I went to bed too late the night before.

c. Groggy and a bit grumpy.

D. I can barely drag myself out of bed. It is very hard to get going.

10. At bedtime, I...

A. Fall asleep pretty easily on most nights.

B. Have a bit of a hard time falling asleep if I have a lot on my mind.

c. Have a hard time settling down. I watch TV or use some electronics.

D. I rely on sleep medications, drugs, or alcohol, and I'm unable to sleep most nights, even if I have to be up the next day.

11. When I eat well and exercise regularly, my weight...

A. Follows the expected course and goes down/ maintains appropriately.

B. Takes longer to come off than I think it should when I eat well and exercise.

c. I have sought out healthcare information because I have a hard time losing/maintaining weight, even when I honestly and faithfully eat healthy and exercise regularly.

D. No matter what I do, I can't lose weight, yet I gain weight very easily.

12. When it comes to making decisions...

A. I weigh the risks/benefits and then decide.

B. I struggle sometimes, especially when I'm tired.

c. I have a hard time, so I either make an impulsive decision or procrastinate.

D. I experience so much difficulty that it's impairing my life or work.

13. My clumsiness and coordination are...
   A. Normal. I make the occasional pratfall.
   B. Hmmm, worse than when I was a kid now that you mention it.
   C. I am running into tables a lot and I'm not nearly as coordinated as I used to be.
   D. I have been accused of being drunk or "on something" (or feel like I am).

14. During cold and flu season...
   A. I get sick every few years.
   B. I get sick every year.
   C. I get sick every few months all year long.
   D. I catch everything that comes along. I'm surprised I haven't gotten Ebola yet.

15. Your skin and face look...
   A. Decent! People are often surprised that I am not younger that I am.
   B. About my actual age.
   C. More wrinkled, eye-bagged, acne-prone, or damaged than other people my age.
   D. Like a person who is older! It is pale, sallow, gray, or generally dull and unhealthy appearing.

16. The thought of taking on a new challenge leaves me...
   A. Excited. Bring it on!
   B. Intrigued...depending on what it is, of course.
   C. Hesitant. What is it and how much work will it be?

    D. Exhausted and looking for the exit.

17. I eat green vegetables...
    A. More than once each day, consistently.
    B. A few times a week.
    C. A few times per month.
    D. Do green M&M's count?

18. I eat fruit...
    A. More than once each day, consistently.
    B. A few times a week.
    C. A few times per month.
    D. Do fruit-flavored Skittles count?

19. I eat fast food (or gas station/on-the-go foods)...
    A. Rarely or never.
    B. A few times per month.
    C. A few times per week.
    D. Daily or multiple times per day.

20. I eat prepackaged meals (e.g., frozen meals, canned meals)...
    A. Rarely or never.
    B. A few times per month.
    C. A few times per week.
    D. Daily or multiple times per day.

21. I eat desserts or sweets...
    A. Rarely or never.
    B. A few times per month.
    C. A few times per week.
    D. Daily or multiple times per day.

22. I overeat or eat even when I'm not hungry...

A. Rarely or never.

B. A few times per month.

C. A few times per week.

D. Daily or multiple times per day.

23. I skip meals or eat one big meal at the end of the day...

A. Rarely.

B. A few times per month.

C. A few times per week.

D. Daily or multiple times per day.

24. I eat while distracted—in front of the TV/electronics, in the car, etc....

A. Rarely.

B. A few times per month.

C. A few times per week.

D. Daily or multiple times per day.

25. I have hidden things I've eaten from others so they won't judge what/how much it is...

A. Rarely.

B. A few times per month.

C. A few times per week.

D. Daily or multiple times per day.

26. I've tried fad diets and weight loss gimmicks...

A. Rarely, if ever. I tend to just eat consistently healthy.

B. I've tried a few with mixed and/or nonsustained results.

C. I have tried several, and my weight tends to yo-yo.

D. I've tried them all, sometimes more than one at

a time. I have no consistent eating style, and my weight is either fluctuating a lot or steadily going up over the years.

27. Your body shape is...
    A. Lean.
    B. Pear-shaped with some excess weight in the hips and legs.
    C. Apple-shaped with excess weight in the abdomen.
    D. Overweight everywhere.

28. Your energy level is...
    A. Pretty good.
    B. Labile and fluctuates with your day/mood/amount of sleep.
    C. Low most of the time.
    D. So low it is interfering with your work and/or quality of life.

29. Your poop
    A. Occurs daily, no issues or concerns.
    B. Is hard or loose, and the frequency is somewhat irregular.
    C. Changes frequently and your bowels feel irritable.
    D. Needs medication (laxatives or bowel stimulants) to even happen.

30. Your pee
    A. Is light yellow and happens multiple times per day.
    B. Is dark and you go a few times a day.
    C. Changes frequently and is unpredictable.

D. Is painful, bloody, or you have had to see a doctor about urinary or kidney problems.

31. You feel anxious, tense, keyed up, stressed, or worried...
    A. Occasionally.
    B. A few times a month.
    C. A few times a week or daily.
    D. So much it is interfering with your life.

32. You feel sad, down, depressed, tearful, or down in the dumps...
    A. Occasionally.
    B. A few times a month.
    C. A few times a week or daily.
    D. So much it is interfering with your life.

33. You feel angry, grumpy, annoyed, frustrated, bitter, or stormy...
    A. Occasionally.
    B. A few times a month.
    C. A few times a week or daily.
    D. So much it is interfering with your life.

34. You feel calm and collected, content, or "chill."
    A. Most days or daily.
    B. A few times a week.
    C. A few times a month.
    D. So rarely you forgot what it is like.

35. You feel happy, joyful, elated, enthusiastic, wonderful, and excited...

A. Most days or daily.

B. A few times a week.

C. A few times a month.

D. So rarely you forgot what it is like.

36. Your exercise routine is...

A. Consistent, at least a few times per week.

B. A few times per month.

C. Occasional and inconsistent.

D. Nonexistent. Both work and leisure are pretty sedentary.

37. If you had to jog a mile right now...

A. It would be no big deal. Sounds fun!

B. It would be difficult, but you could do it.

C. You would have to walk part/most of it.

D. You likely couldn't finish a mile, even with walking.

38. How many push-ups can you do right now? (Feel free to try it!)

A. Twenty or more.

B. Ten (but maybe need a break).

C. Can't do ten, even with the modification on my knees.

D. Probably one or two.

39. How often do you do active hobbies, such as swimming, dancing, fast walking, biking, hiking, heavy yardwork/cleaning, or other things that get you out of breath?

A. A few times per week or more.

B. A few times per month.

C. A few times per year.

D. I don't really do these things.

40. How is your balance?

   A. I could easily walk on a balance beam without help, maybe do a spin or two.

   B. I'm fine on the ground, no issues.

   C. I sometimes need to hold on to things or have difficulty changing direction quickly.

   D. I often bump into things, have fallen more than once, or rely on a cane or walker to get around safely.

ACKNOWLEDGMENTS

I am filled with gratitude for so many wonderful people who have had a positive influence on my life. I could fill thousands of pages with love and appreciation for each and every one of these people. However, those who know me also know I'm a huge tree hugger, so in the interest of space, I will try to be brief.

To my parents: Thanks for giving me life! I'm sure the whole birthing thing was a lot of work (at least for Mom!)—not to mention the whole raising me part. You say it takes eighteen years to raise a baby human, but now that I'm in my thirties, you know that never ends, right?! Your ongoing guidance, friendship, support, and love are amazing!

Mom: Thank you for being there for me even when it isn't easy. You will give me a (loving) butt-kicking and amazing encouragement whenever I need it. You are the queen of amazing ideas, a badass grandma, and someone I'm so lucky to call a friend. You always, always answer the call (and you are my number-one draft pick for the zombie apocalypse).

Dad: Thank you for being my calm, steady rock. You love me and encourage me no matter what. You even drove me to a speaking engagement when I was pregnant and vomiting and sat there through my entire ACLS talk, which was probably pretty boring if you don't need to know much about the finer points of defibrillation. You always have a kind word and a hug. You are my triceps hero, my constant source of "keen grasp of the obvious," and my safe place—and I appreciate that!

To my siblings: Thanks for being my partners in crime and for not locking me in a closet forever like you threatened to do! I know both of you probably would have rather had a dog than a baby sister, but since you were stuck with me, I hope it mostly didn't suck. Dad wouldn't have let you get a dog anyway, so there!

Kelly: You are my PD power sister! Thanks for sharing a birthday with me...like you had a choice, haha! We even survived sharing a room, and you didn't snuff me out in my sleep! From a masking-tape divider in our room to best friends, we've come a long way! I can't imagine my life without my big sister birthday buddy. I love my sista!

Roger: Thank you for being the kind of brother who harasses me and makes me laugh and loves me forever, even though I'm better looking (haha). I still haven't forgotten that you used to try to scare guys away so I could never date (although a few of them deserved to be scared away, lol). Thanks for being there through thick and thin. Having a best friend that shares blood is badass.

Grandma: You are a badass grandma. Remember when we did shots in Mexico with some Canadian tourists and you led a conga line around the bar? You are fun and loving, and I appreciate you sharing your life with me. Thank you for allowing me to speak to your club. You are an amazing encourager and a great listener.

Doug: Remember that time you told me that you thought I should write a book? Little did you know I had one inside of me already. Thank you for encouraging me to let it out. I am so grateful to you for so many things, but most of all for your support and kind words. I am your number-one fan for the healthy changes you've made, and I look forward to many healthy years to come!

Bobbie: I miss you every day. Unlike most sitcom characters, I actually got to have a mother-in-law whom I loved. You were crazy, talented, caring, perpetually late, incredibly generous, and uniquely you. I tried so hard to live up to what I thought an ideal daughter-in-law should be, and you never stopped reminding me that you loved me just the way I was. I know you would be so proud of me for chasing my dreams.

To the **McKennons, Roberts, Neubachers, Stuefs, Kriegs, Parkers, Hopes,** and all of my extended family: I love and appreciate you so very much. Thank you for helping create who I am and cheering me on for who I can be.

Leslie Frick: I don't know how the stars aligned so you could come into our lives, but I will always be grateful. You are truly an angel in every way. I absolutely love you, and I learn as much from you as the kids do. Thank you for becoming family!

Dawn Gaden: My counselor and coach extraordinaire, thank you for helping keep my mind healthy so I am able to help others. You have helped me help myself in so many ways and I cannot express enough appreciation for the valuable role you play in my life. (www.dawngaden-therapy.com)

I have some of the most amazing friends on the planet, a loving and supportive tribe of people who will always have my back and care about me (even when I wear bad fashion!). You helped me when I was sick and at my lowest and cheer me on when I'm at my best. **Cathy and Solomon Knicely, Donna Helms, Amy Smark-Gorgas, Abi Brackney, Stan Leong, Sema Contreas, Cindy Weintraub, Camelia Eljawad, Cathy and Vytau Virskus,** and the **Virskus** clan. Thank you for your encouragement and for sticking with me when I spread my wings and go off the beaten path. I am beyond grateful to call you friends.

I believe in finding your tribe, and I belong to some of the best! To my Facebook tribes that support me, teach me, and meme me—**EMDOCS** and **The PMG**—my life would not be the same without you! Thank you Vanitha, Hala, K Kay, Stephen, Dominic, Joe, Howie, Drora, Katydid, Chu, and all of my favorite "irregulars," as well as the rest of the mama docs/BAFERD tribes. Sending much love!

To my **Beaumont** family: working in the trenches isn't for the faint of heart. What we do, other people can't imagine, and having each other's backs makes anything bearable. I've worked with some truly amazing people over the past thirteen-plus years, and I am honored to be part of the team.

There are many people who have helped teach me, influence me, guide me, and open doors for me. I never cease to be amazed and incredibly grateful to the people who have helped and mentored me in my growth process.

CM: You taught me an incredible amount of things, both directly and indirectly. Your influence on me persists, and I appreciate all of the work/PD/life lessons. Thank you for introducing me to a whole new world. I will always be grateful for the start you gave me. Thank you for being a part of my journey.

Victoria Lucia, PhD: Thank you for letting me guerilla my way into your "Promotion and Maintenance of Health" course. It has been the most amazing and fun opportunity to get to teach Behavior Change and Motivational Interviewing to medical students. You have been supportive, helpful, encouraging, loving, directive, and have given me sufficient freedom to be my crazy, authentic self. I hope to teach these courses forever! Thank you for letting me in the door.

Dara Kass, MD: Holy shit! I meant it when I said you changed my life! Thank you for giving me a microphone and a chance. I always knew I had it in me, and you gave me my first big break. The FEMinEM video you made of my "Confidence and Imposter Syndrome" talk helped open doors for me, and I will be forever grateful to you for my start. Thank you for allowing it to be released into the wild (haha, YouTube). The movement that you have started will continue to bring awesomeness to the world. You are a role model and a badass, and I will be a FEMinEM for life! (www.feminem.org)

To Miz, Rob-O, Aaron, Paul, Tom and the team at **HIPPO** (www.hippoed.com): Thank you for welcoming me as a guest! I am so passionate about teaching and getting to work with the best team and med ed is a dream come true!

Mizuho Spangler, MD: You advocated for me and had my back! I owe my stage spot to you! You are my role model and hero, the kind of woman who reaches out and helps elevate other women. You are a badass educator, mom, and doctor, and I love that I get to call you friend. (www.threemommydoctors.com)

Verne Harnish: Thank you for seeing my potential. You took me under your wing and helped me fly. I will never forget sitting at a tiki bar in Florida with you and sketching out the ideas for this very book on a napkin—in the rain, no less! You are the king of Scaling Up, a talented and dynamic speaker, an excellent author, a genuinely nice and caring friend, and an incredibly well-traveled and interesting person. I am grateful to know you! (www.gazelles.com)

Joe Polish: I hardly know where to even begin. You are one of the most extraordinary humans and I am beyond grateful for having you in my life. I've heard you speak a ton of times, and I never get tired of you sharing your wisdom and awesomeness. I love quoting you in my book and in my talks; you say really smart shit! You really truly make the world a better place, and you know I admire the crap out of you! I am honored to support you on your personal mission to change the conversation about how we view and treat addicts (and anyone fighting silent battles!) with compassion instead of judgment. Thank you for being an amazing human, and thank you for becoming my dear friend. You are the kind of person I will always answer the phone for. (www.JoePolish.com)

Eunice and the entire **Genius Network** crew: So much awesomeness in one group of people! You have always been so kind and welcoming of me—you make me feel like family! I love you dearly! This mastermind group is so much more than I ever imagined! (www.geniusnetwork.com)

Sean Stephenson: Speaking master and guru, thank you for helping me grow! You help bring out the best in people (even when you have to poke them with a stick!). You are hilarious, incredibly talented, and a wonderful inspiration (I would clap for you if you robbed a bank, lol!)! I look forward to watching your **Lucrative Speaker** brand grow, although no one can captivate an audience like you can! (www.seanstephenson.com)

Joel Weldon: I adore your positive attitude and energy! You have given me so much kindness and encouragement and wisdom. You have taken my good talks and helped them to be great. You are unsurpassed in your expertise; you truly are the **Ultimate Speaker**. I look forward to seeing you improve the world of public speaking for everyone! (www.successcomesincans.com)

Jason Fladlien: Thank you for being there for me. Knowing you are on the other end of a text or a call brings a smile to my face every time. I appreciate your advice and encouragement as I drag myself (sometimes kicking and screaming, lol) into becoming an entrepreneur. Everything you touch turns to gold, so if you could pick this book and shake it a few times and sprinkle magic on it, that would be great! Also, my memes are funnier than your jokes. (www.rapidcrush.com)

Julie Gandolfo: Thank you for being my meditation guru! You are a shining light, and I appreciate the peace you have brought into my life! You are my soul sister, and I love you! (www.waveofblissmeditation.com)

Jeff Madoff: Thank you for the many wonderful conversations; I could talk to you for hours! Your play, *Mr. Personality*, blew me away. I can't wait to see it shared with the world. Speaking of sharing, thank you for introducing me to your very talented children! **Jake Madoff** has done an amazing job on my website, and **Audrey Madoff** is an outstanding graphic designer! What a fantastic family!

It is hard to believe that I have had the opportunity to meet some of my absolute favorite authors in person:

David Osborn, author of *Wealth Can't Wait* and *The Miracle Morning for Millionaires* (www.davidosborn.com): You are an awesome guy, and I love your insights and wisdom! Thank you for your guidance and kindness! It has been amazing to have the opportunity to learn from you and get to know you. I look forward to many more wonderful conversations!

Hal Elrod (www.halelrod.com), author of the *Miracle Morning* series of books (and more!): You are such a great guy, husband, and father! I had a great time seeing the Cirque show with you, getting organic juice (remember the fireman shot?!), and hanging out with your family. It was an honor to be in Sedona for the premier of the *Miracle Morning* movie! You and Ursula and the kids are great—wishing you nothing but the best! You are winning at everything, especially family!

Anna David: Damn girl, you are killing it! You are a best-selling author, Light Hustler, and a definite hottie! I love getting to hang out with you any time I can. Your books, podcasts, television appearances, and a million other things are amazing! Keep changing the world. I'll always be a fan! (www.annadavid.com)

Benjamin Hardy: You are just as genuine, nice, and intelligent in person as you are in your books. I've loved the opportunity to share many conversations and meals with you. *Willpower Doesn't Work* is an amazing book, so amazing that I use it in my teaching at our medical school! Your writing on www.medium.com is unsurpassed. Keep bringing your awesomeness into the world! (www.benjaminhardy.com)

J.P. Sears (www.awakenwithjp.com): You are one of the most hilarious and insightful people I've had the pleasure of meeting. Your wit and delivery are freaking amazing, and your YouTube videos are the best, and everyone needs to watch them! I really enjoy the positivity and love you bring to the world. I adore you and Amber, and I look forward to your future books and shows. Keep being Ultra Spiritual!

To the authors I love and admire and hope one day to meet: **Jen Sincero, Rory Vaden, Brian Tracy, Marshall Goldsmith, Melissa Ambrosini, Amy Cuddy, Angela Duckworth, Charles Duhigg, Carol Dweck, Chip and Dan Heath, Dan Sullivan, Robert Cialdini, Steven Pressfield, Kamal Ravikant, Vishen Lakhiani, Gary John Bisshop, Mel Robbins, Sheryl Sandberg, Dr. Michael Gregor,** and **Adele Faber and Elaine Mazlish.** And here's to **Zig Ziglar** for making this world better for having lived in it!

To the **Scribe** crew: Thank you for all of your hard work. **Emily**, you are so kind and encouraging, I wish we lived in the same area! Thank you for keeping the project on task! (I want to read *your* book some day!) **John**, thank you for the hours on the phone where you took all of my knowledge and passion and helped turn it into something organized! And **Chas**, for the hours upon hours: I've spoken to you more on the phone than anyone else in the past few years! You made me feel comfortable and open and helped draw out the best in me. You help me find the best words to express all of the excitement and passion in my mind. You let me wander into (many!) tangents and sometimes find the diamonds in the randomness. You do a good job setting limits in an encouraging way (or this book would have hundreds more exclamation points, lol!!) and your guidance as a grammar Gandhi should be shared with the masses. You are my partner and friend in the process and I can't wait to work on *Resilience* with you! **Scribe**: I could not have done this book without the most amazing team in the business. Thank you!

And finally, to **Ryan**: Where to even begin? There are not enough words for all the things and stuff. You are my polar bear and lobster. I'm so proud of *your* accomplishments. You are amazing, and I appreciate more things than I can count. But if I had to try to count, it would be infinity. Plus we made some pretty amazing little humans.

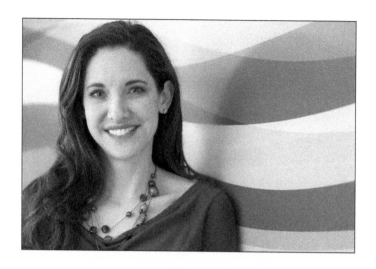

ABOUT THE
AUTHOR

JAIME HOPE, MD, is a dual board-certified physician working outside of Detroit, Michigan, in one of the busiest emergency departments in the country. In over twelve years on the job, she has learned that no matter what brought her patients to the ER, they all want the same thing: to live happier, healthier lives. Today, whether she's helping patients, teaching future doctors, or engaging the local community, Dr. Hope is showing others how to create better habits and make healthy living fun, practical, and accessible.

CPSIA information can be obtained
at www.ICGtesting.com
Printed in the USA
BVHW030214100119
537513BV00003B/9/P